INED Population Studies

Volume 6

This book series is devoted to publications of international relevance in population studies and demography as promoted by the French National Institute for Demographic Studies (INED, Paris). As one social science among many, demography is interlinked with related disciplines such as sociology, anthropology, history or linguistics, and continuously explores its boundaries with neighbouring disciplines, ranging from epidemiology and biology to economics. The studies published in this series are based on solid empirical research and firm methodological foundations or research fi ndings. Particular attention is paid to long-term and/or collaborative surveys. The series provides international visibility to works of high academic standard, and promotes an internationally acknowledged style of demographic research, upheld by INED for more than half a century and rekindled in various fi elds such as the study of demographic situations around the world, the relationship between demographic conditions and development; international comparisons; migration, identities and territories; family studies; gender studies and sexuality; ageing, health and mortality; trajectories, mobility and social networks.

More information about this series at http://www.springer.com/series/11579

Catherine Bonvalet • Éva Lelièvre
Editors

Family Beyond Household and Kin

Life Event Histories and Entourage, a French Survey

Springer

Editors
Catherine Bonvalet
INED
Paris, France

Éva Lelièvre
INED
Paris, France

Original French edition, *De la famille à l''entourage*, published by INED, 2012, Coll. "Grandes Enquêtes"

ISSN 2214-2452 ISSN 2214-2460 (electronic)
INED Population Studies
ISBN 978-3-319-24682-6 ISBN 978-3-319-24684-0 (eBook)
DOI 10.1007/978-3-319-24684-0

Library of Congress Control Number: 2015958788

Springer Cham Heidelberg New York Dordrecht London

Printed on acid-free paper

Springer International Publishing AG Switzerland is part of Springer Science+Business Media (www.springer.com)

Acknowledgements

This book continues a long tradition of research on housing and the family at the French Institute for Demographic Studies (INED). It follows in the footsteps of Alfred Sauvy, Louis Henry, Guy Pourcher, and Daniel Courgeau for housing and mobility and of Louis Roussel, Catherine Villeneuve-Gokalp, and Hervé Le Bras for the family.

This research would not have been possible without close collaboration between researchers and institutional partners who contributed to the scientific project through their financial support for the *Biographies et entourage* survey.

Launching a major survey takes years of preparation and involves a large number of people. We are especially grateful to the 178 interviewers and team members who took charge of fieldwork, coding, and data cleansing with the support of the INED Surveys department. The high quality of the survey data reflects the long-term dedication of a survey team that included many technical and administrative staff, PhD students, and internees.

We are also grateful to the translators, Madeleine Grieve and Oliver Waine, and give our special thanks to Catriona Dutreuilh who organized and oversaw the translation of the whole book into English.

We also wish to thank all the organizations which provided funding for the project (CNAF – Caisse Nationale d'Allocations Familiales; CNAV – Caisse Nationale d'Assurance Vieillesse; DPM – Direction de la Population et des Migrations; DREES – Direction de la recherche, des études, de l'évaluation et des statistiques; DREIF – Direction Régionale de l'Équipement d'Île-de-France; IAURIF – Institut d'Aménagement et d'Urbanisme de la Région Île-de-France; ODEP Mairie de Paris – Observatoire du Développement Économique Parisien; RATP – Régie Autonome des Transports Parisiens; Ministère de la Recherche; Action Concertée Incitative Ville).

Acknowledgements

Contents

Contents

Contributors

Catherine Bonvalet Institut national d'études démographiques (INED), Paris, France

Céline Clément Centre de recherches sociologiques et politiques de Paris (Cresppa-GTM), Université Paris Ouest Nanterre La Défense, Nanterre, France

Valérie Golaz Institut national d'études démographiques (INED), Paris, France

Marianne Kempeneers Département de sociologie, Université de Montréal (UdM), Quebec, Canada

Éva Lelièvre Institut national d'études démographiques (INED), Paris, France

Christine Tichit UR 1303 Alimentation et sciences sociales (ALISS), Institut national de recherches agronomiques (INRA), Paris, France

Géraldine Vivier Institut national d'études démographiques (INED), Paris, France

Chapter 1
The Family Beyond Household and Kin, Introducing the *Entourage*

Catherine Bonvalet and Éva Lelièvre

Since the 1990s, large surveys have been conducted on relationships and exchanges within families in many European countries (Bonvalet and Ogg 2007). At the forefront of family research in demography, after the "golden years" of the nuclear family as sole reference, interest is now focusing on documenting the entire range of familial living arrangements – living apart together, stepfamilies, living with significant others, new extended families, etc. – which raises new questions on the role of the family, on the nature of exchanges and on family configurations. The wider family group, with its potential ability to offset the impact of economic crises, has been attracting growing attention, particularly in a context of rising unemployment, housing shortage and population ageing. Family ties and other forms of social capital appear to be key to understanding families as configurations. One way to approach wider family groups which extend beyond a single household is to consider their territory.

In this respect, the study of associated dwellings and neighbourhoods has proven a particularly fertile terrain for observing the family beyond the household and examining kinship ties in urban contexts (Young and Willmott 1957). Moreover, given the changes in the family observed since the 1970s and the fact that its sphere of influence extends well beyond the household (with children of divorced parents living in both their parents' homes, couples living apart together and stepfamilies, for example), this perspective is especially effective for identifying the factors at play in the private realm. Studying how spatial mobility is associated with the dynamics of affinity sheds light on the relationships that people maintain with their *entourage*, in other words, the way in which the *family organizes its territories* through its concentration in one place or, conversely, its dispersal in spatial terms. It also provides new clues to identifying the residential and urban dynamics at work at the macro level (Bonvalet et al. 2007). Through a joint analysis of family organization and residential choices, it is possible to move beyond a purely instrumental vision

C. Bonvalet (✉) • É. Lelièvre (✉)
Institut national d'études démographiques (INED), Paris, France
e-mail: bonvalet@ined.fr; eva@ined.fr

C. Bonvalet, É. Lelièvre (eds.), *Family Beyond Household and Kin*,
INED Population Studies 6, DOI 10.1007/978-3-319-24684-0_1

of the family and housing and consequently to change the way in which both are studied and considered. On the one hand, a family-oriented approach allows for a better understanding of households' residential and property-related behaviours, while an approach based on residential mobility proves useful in revealing the motives associated with the affinities and obligations between the family members.

The *Biographies et entourage* survey combines a relational approach and an event history approach. It is based on the premise that the nuclear family (or the household) can only be truly understood when considered within its wider network, and that the situation at a given moment is the result of past residential and family histories of all family members. Over their life course, individuals modify both their ties and their location, and the family spatial configuration reflects a balance of distance and closeness which partly depends on relationships within the circle of family and friends. Reconciling the household and the family, the concept of *entourage* broadens the individual's reference group to include the network of parents, siblings, co-residing and non-co-residing children, spouses and their parents, all the people with whom the individual has lived at some point in his/her life and any other person who, whether related or not, has played a key role in their lives.

The *Biographies et entourage* survey was conducted in 2001 by the French Institute for Demographic Studies (INED) among a representative sample of residents of Paris and the surrounding Île-de-France region born between 1930 and 1950. Its aim was to follow changes in the respondents' *entourage* over their life course by reconstituting its composition, its geographic distribution and the level of co-residence between members. It is also possible to reconstruct the territorial boundaries and the succession of roles played in the network and their evolution over time; people interviewed having each been a grandchild, a child, a parent and, in turn, possibly a grandparent.

Mobilizing the concept of *entourage*, the survey first sought to collect information on individuals' networks of sociability beyond the household and family ties, and to understand how these networks function; second, as a life event history survey, the data include records of the family, residential and occupational trajectories not just of respondents but also, for the first time, of the members of respondents' entourages, hence the plural ("*Biographie s*") in the title. It is thus possible to update longitudinal indicators (not produced by any other surveys) for recent birth cohorts, concerning, for example, the average number of dwellings, jobs and unions that individuals have had, for birth cohorts born between 1930 and 1950, bearing in mind that this information was provided by respondents aged 50 and over. These indicators, combined with a significant quantity of additional information, provide details of residential and occupational mobility and family histories that complement respondents' mobility trajectories and, more generally, their individual trajectories.

This book brings together a sample of the many studies conducted on the basis of the survey. Half of the chapters from the French book "*De la famille à l'entourage*" were selected, in agreement with Springer, to focus the publication on the stimulating concept of the *entourage*, starting with a presentation of the concept, followed by chapters focusing on data collection and analysis.

Chapter 2 gives a detailed presentation of the survey, its genesis and goals. It traces its genealogy via two channels – life event history surveys on residential mobility, and surveys on family networks and networks of solidarity – thus revealing the combination of conceptual and empirical approaches which led to the design of the survey. This is followed by a practical description of the steps involved in fine-tuning the survey questions, choosing the data-collection universes, selecting the sample population and processing the collected data.

Chapter 3 is a translation of the initial article published in 1995 in which we presented the concept of *entourage* for the first time. This chapter highlights the need for a concept to capture the dynamics of the reference groups to which individuals belong throughout their lives, and justifies the use of a new notion: the *entourage*, which includes the members of the successive households to which a given individual has belonged, together with family members and other key individuals designated by the respondent. Subsequent chapters describe the entourages of respondents at different points in their life histories.

Chapters 4 and 5 reveal the rich and varied nature of parental entourages during respondents' childhoods. These include not only the socially instituted parental figures, well established in the field of demography, but also *de facto* parental figures comprising individuals who have played a complementary role, sometimes replacing a respondent's biological or adoptive mother or father. The composition of the family-based entourage in the course of respondents' lives is presented in greater detail in Chap. 5, in which the authors compare the various configurations, with respondents' appraisals of the periods in question.

Chapter 6 focuses on respondents' relationships with their elderly parents and confirms the pivotal role of respondents aged 50–70 in the family network. The post-war baby-boomer birth cohorts have not – despite the fears of some in the early 1970s[1] – disengaged from the family sphere. On the contrary, they are strongly committed to family life, supporting their ageing parents, helping their children – whose entry into adulthood has taken place in completely different conditions from theirs – and above all fully embracing their role as grandparents. This is clear in Chap. 7, which examines the changing place of grandparents using data from the quantitative survey and complemented by an analysis of the qualitative interviews conducted as part of the survey.

Chapter 8 then considers families' territories based on the specific cases of stepfamilies. This chapter highlights the permanence of certain locations throughout complex family trajectories, based on a qualitative study conducted as part of the *Biographies et entourage* survey. The question of stepfamilies is approached from the standpoint of how dwellings are shared or divided between the family members that frequent them, highlighting notions of permanence and rupture in an original way.

Chapter 9 examines the places associated with the family and the territory within which family relations are organized. Considering places frequented by respondents, places of origin and places defined by the homes of family members brings to light a set of different territories, extending beyond the confines of the Paris region. They define a "geography" of the family which sums up its migration history and reveals the organization of family ties.

---

[1] Cooper D., 1970, *The Death of the Family*, Pantheon Books, 145 p.

Finally, Chap. 10 concludes with a discussion of the methodological challenges raised by the study dynamics of "family solidarity". The value of the *Biographies et entourage* survey for studying the different temporal aspects of exchanges is examined, in comparison with an extensive array of other quantitative surveys.

The notion of household has proved inadequate for capturing changes in the family. By exploring the limits of this notion, which led to the development of new concepts, such as that of the *entourage*, this book shows that it is possible to build theoretical tools and to design surveys that capture the realities of the group of family and significant others who accompany individuals throughout their life course. As couples adopt new modes of cohabitation, as family trajectories become ever more complex and as increasing life expectancy at advanced ages means that families now often include three or even four generations of adults, the family can no longer be defined in terms of a shared roof. Today, it is the existence of strong ties beyond the household, and no longer the walls of the house, that defines the family contours forming the *entourage*.

References

Bonvalet, C., & Ogg, J. (Eds.). (2007). *Measuring family support in Europe*. London: Southern Universities Press.

Bonvalet, C., Gotman, A., & Grafmeyer, Y. (Eds.). (2007). *Family kindship and place in France*. London: Southern Universities Press/Ined.

Young, M., & Willmott, P. (1957). *Family and kinship in East London*. London: Routledge and Kegan Paul.

Chapter 2
Presentation of the *Biographies et entourage* Survey

Catherine Bonvalet and Éva Lelièvre

Since 1970, lifestyles have changed radically and families have diversified and changed with them. The family unit has evolved within a geographically variable space that needs to be understood, as it is this space, and not just housing alone, that defines the family. Today, in a context of separations, reconstituted families and multi-residence, the family extends far beyond the four walls of the home. These developments have led researchers in the field to extend their investigations to the interpersonal relationships constructed throughout people's lives, and to the spaces in which these relationships take place. This approach has called for new observation tools and new concepts that are better suited to describing the realities and dynamics of family life in time and space. More specifically, a long-term study was deemed an essential condition for meeting the challenge at hand, namely to describe the network of close family and friends – which we shall refer to hereafter as the "entourage" – who are present throughout an individual's life, and the nature of this network in spatial terms; and to do so in such a way as to identify what constitutes a "system" from both a family standpoint and a residential standpoint. Another key consideration today – 20 years after the *Triple biographie* (Triple event history) survey, and 10 years after the *Proches et parents* (Close friends and relatives) survey – is the need for updated knowledge regarding residential mobility and kinship. It was in order to respond to these two objectives that the *Biographies et entourage* (Life-event histories and entourage) survey was conducted by INED in 2000–2001. By gathering information about the family histories, residential histories and occupational histories of 2830 residents of Île-de-France (the Paris region) and their entourages, this survey sought to provide a more detailed analysis of individual trajectories in order to assess the influence of close family and friends on individual choices, and vice versa.

C. Bonvalet (✉) • É. Lelièvre (✉)
Institut national d'études démographiques (INED), Paris, France
e-mail: bonvalet@ined.fr; eva@ined.fr

C. Bonvalet, É. Lelièvre (eds.), *Family Beyond Household and Kin*,
INED Population Studies 6, DOI 10.1007/978-3-319-24684-0_2

By combining two approaches – one based on relationships, the other on life events – the *Biographies et entourage* survey sought to collect the data necessary to describe and analyse the family network and its role throughout an individual's life. To achieve this, it was necessary to move away from conventional representations of certain concepts such as the household or the primary residence, and instead put forward new versions of them, such as the notion of the "entourage" on the one hand and that of the residential system on the other. It was also necessary to take account of the contexts in which individual trajectories, operating at multiple levels (individual, family, social, etc.), take place. None of these levels is mutually exclusive, each following its own rhythm and pattern of change. This contextualization would enable the study of relational interactions that change over respondents' lifetimes by combining individual, historical and intergenerational temporalities (Kempeneers et al. 2007).

In order to test the feasibility of such an approach, preliminary work was conducted in the 1990s, based on a joint analysis of the *Peuplement et dépeuplement de Paris* (Population and depopulation of Paris) and *Triple biographie* surveys. It is through this work that the concept of the entourage emerged, together with ideas on how data relating to this concept could be collected and analysed. In this way, the conceptual groundwork was laid and the first tests of the notion of "entourage" were carried out. The results of these tests were initially presented to a symposium in Canada (Bonvalet and Lelièvre 1995a) before being formalized in a collective article (Lelièvre et al. 1997) published just as the first qualitative explorations were beginning.

For this reason, in addition to conventional objectives such as updating knowledge on residential mobility, geographical trajectories and the family network, one of the key aims of the *Biographies et entourage* survey was to examine and analyse these concepts, and measure how useful they were in order to better gauge the influence of the entourage on individual trajectories throughout an individual's lifetime.

Before proceeding with the presentation of the survey itself, we felt it would be useful to show how *Biographies et entourage* is related to other INED surveys[1] – which is not to say that it has not benefited from the contributions of other French and international research; the point of restricting ourselves to the work of INED is to highlight the direct ancestry of the *Biographies et entourage* survey.

[1] The *Biographies et entourage* survey has benefited from the contributions made by other studies with no links to INED; its international heritage is extensively retraced in the recently republished work by GRAB (*Groupe de réflexion sur l'approche biographique*) titled *Biographies d'enquêtes* (GRAB 2009). Nevertheless, it must be emphasized that only large institutions such as INED and INSEE (the French National Institute for Statistics and Economic Studies) have the necessary resources to conduct long-term studies. In France, Françoise Cribier's work (1990, 1992) on mobility among several generations of Parisians remains an exception.

2.1 Genealogy of the *Biographies et entourage* Survey

The *Biographies et entourage* survey was designed to collect information needed to comprehend the family group beyond the household alone, as well as the residential space in which the family group develops and changes in the long term. The conditions for observing and monitoring respondents' entourages have a dual heritage, as the *Biographies et entourage* survey is situated at the intersection of two series of surveys conducted by INED since the 1960s: surveys on residential mobility and surveys on the family and networks (Fig. 2.1).

2.1.1 The Legacy of Surveys on Mobility and Residential Trajectories[2]

Mobility, like fertility and mortality, is a demographic phenomenon whose analysis has always been the subject of research by INED. Indeed, from its creation in 1945, when its remit was to study population-related issues in all their forms, the work of France's new demographic institute focused in particular on the themes of internal migration and housing, which were of vital importance in the post-war years. Demographic studies produced on these subjects by INED quickly stood out for the originality of their approaches. In 1946, Alfred Sauvy published an article titled *Logement et population* (Housing and Population), in which he explained that the main reasons for the housing shortage and the slump in the construction industry were linked not just to rent-control measures enacted in 1914, but also to the ageing of the population and a drop in birth rates. It was his view that a housing policy should be an instrument for correcting demographic imbalances, and that INED should conduct in-depth surveys on this theme. This led to the production of two types of study in the 1950s: the first sought to analyse the demand for housing among the French population via surveys[3] and monographs, while the second attempted, at the initiative of Louis Henry, to identify housing needs using projections (Henry 1949, 1950). In 1959, the number of housing units built since the end of the war reached the golden figure of 320,000 deemed necessary to meet the needs of French households and respond to a rising birth rate following the baby boom (reversing a previous downward trend). The primary concern then was no longer to incite the government to build new housing. Instead, another problem was beginning to emerge in France, namely a rural exodus and migration to the major cities.

[2]This section on INED's series of "mobility" surveys is based on the review of urban research produced by INED since its creation in 1945, edited by Catherine Bonvalet, titled *Logement, mobilité et populations urbaines* (Paris, CNRS Éditions, "Cahiers du PIR Villes" collection, 1994).

[3]In particular the survey by Alain Girard and Jean Stoetzel on the desires of the French with regard to housing and their place of residence (1945), the survey on the housing of young households in the former Seine *département* (which covered Paris and its inner suburbs) (Girard and Bastide 1952), and the survey on lodging houses (*hôtels meublés*) in Paris (Michel 1955).

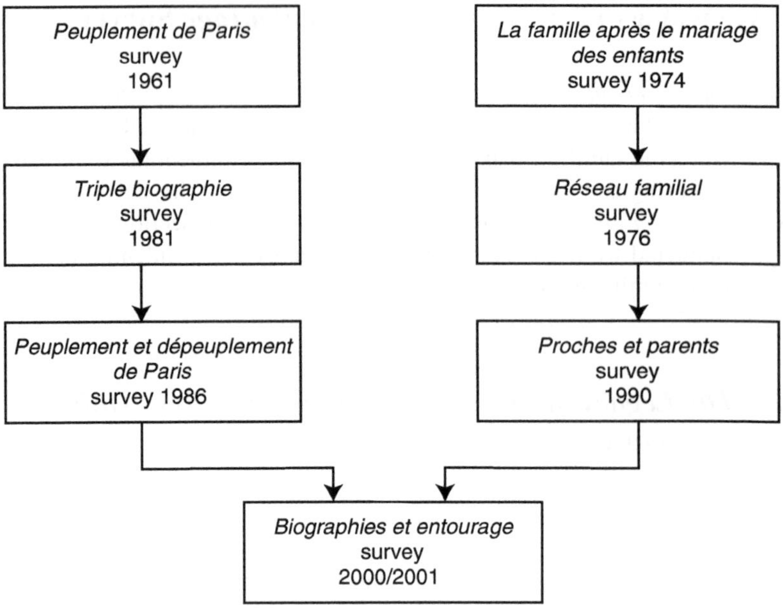

Fig. 2.1 Genealogy of the *Biographies et entourage* survey

Furthermore, the subsequent increase in the urban population was to play a role in highlighting the housing issue in new contexts, such as the growth of large urban areas, and of the Paris urban area in particular. The watchwords were urban planning and the study of internal migration and rural exodus.

It was in this context that INED initiated two major mobility surveys in 1961. The first concerned population growth in Paris, while the second focused on migration within the provinces.

Research gradually moved from a migration-based approach (e.g. rural exodus, development of large urban areas) to the analysis of relationships between forms of mobility and demographic behaviour, and then later to life-event history analysis. The series of surveys on mobility comprises three major studies: *Peuplement de Paris* (Population growth in Paris) (1961), *Triple biographie* (1981) and *Peuplement et dépeuplement de Paris* (1986).

2.1.1.1 The *Peuplement de Paris* and *Mobilité géographique et concentration en France* Surveys

In the analysis of urbanization and migration, Paris is a special case. Its growth can be explained by very high levels of inward migration: according to Paul Clerc (1967), net immigration between 1954 and 1962 represented 70,000–80,000 people per year. Ever since the work of Bertillon (1894), Parisians' origins have aroused the curiosity of researchers and, as early as 1950, Louis Chevalier wrote a book on the subject titled *Formation de la population parisienne au XIX*[e] *siècle* (Formation of the Parisian population in the 19th century). Guy Pourcher continued this research on the basis of the *Peuplement de Paris* survey (1961) and study the geographical origins of migrants, their family origins, and their geographical mobility based on the number of times they changed residence. The conditions surrounding their arrival in Paris and the reasons for their migration to the capital, together with their mobility within the urban area and their intentions to move, were analysed, thus revealing migrants' capacity for integrating into the Parisian population: once they had arrived in Paris, little distinguished them from Parisians, be it in terms of their fertility levels, their location within the urban area, or their housing. While they differed with regard to their background of origin (owing to the prevalence of farming), their occupational mobility was similar to that of Parisians.

The vast majority of migrants were very satisfied with their residential mobility, even if they had experienced accommodation difficulties when they first arrived because of a shortage of housing. Guy Pourcher noted that migrants continued to perpetuate the migratory process by returning frequently to their region of origin and by attracting young people from the provinces to the capital where mutual support networks were well established: half of all migrants had a close friend or relative who already lived in the Paris area (Pourcher 1963, 1964).

The second survey, *Mobilité géographique et concentration en France* (Geographical mobility and concentration in France), conducted in provincial France, complemented the Parisian survey to a certain extent and sought to compare mobility towards Paris with mobility within other regions of France. Were the reasons that motivated people from the provinces to "go up to the capital" the same as those that led people from the provinces to move from one town to another, or from a village to a big city (Pourcher et al. 1964)? The authors highlighted one very interesting result in particular: the reasons for mobility changed according to the size of the town or city. Occupational mobility mainly concerned town- and city-dwellers, while matrimonial mobility primarily concerned rural areas. The reasons for migration to large cities were the same as those mentioned in the Parisian survey (Pourcher 1966). Specifically, there seemed to be a cycle of changes of residence: at the start of the life cycle, the reasons were mainly family-related, with marriage and the arrival of children, later becoming occupational, and then once again family-related following retirement.

But mobility and change did not go hand in hand with ignorance about the destinations people were headed for. In fact, "most of the time, [such moves were] not an adventure or a leap into the unknown": migration was to a certain extent experienced not so much as a break with one's living environment of origin as a reunion in a new living environment. For Bastide and Girard, mobility meant not "the disintegration of the family but, on the contrary, the reconstitution of the family in the place of arrival".[4]

---

[4] We shall return to this significant result in the section on the series of surveys on the family, as it was reported at a time marked by the theories of Talcott Parsons (1955), who suggested that the nuclear family, defined as parents and children only, and thus highly mobile (as it is free from any other attachments), was the only form of family suited to industrial society.

It was on the basis of this second survey that Guy Pourcher carried out the first analysis of generational mobility, applying analytical methods identical to those that had been developed by Louis Henry for fertility. The aim was to describe the geographical mobility of individuals in each birth cohort and try to assess the scale of occupational changes that typically accompanied changes of residence (Pourcher 1966). In Guy Pourcher's view, retrospective observation was altogether appropriate for long-term analysis. Respondents were asked about their successive dwellings and the different occupations in which they had worked. On the basis of these data, he calculated mobility rates for each generational group by determining the ratio of first moves at each age to the numbers of individuals concerned in each cohort. The highest rate was found between the ages of 20 and 24, before rapidly falling thereafter. The sum of these mobility rates thus gave the mean number of moves for each cohort.

The results of this analysis clearly showed the value of long-term analysis: the cohorts where mobility was lowest were those born between 1881 and 1885, as they reached adulthood around the time of the First World War. By contrast, cohorts born between 1896 and 1900 had a higher level of mobility following the economic recovery after 1918, and those born between the turn of the twentieth century and 1914 were less mobile owing to the economic crisis of the 1930s. While occupational mobility (calculated on the basis of job changes) accelerated from one cohort to another, changes in social status remained rare. Pourcher was therefore the first person to use long-term analysis in the study of occupational and residential mobility; on average, the oldest cohorts of his sample underwent 1.7 changes of residence and 0.34 occupational changes. However, Pourcher would have liked to go further in his analysis of the relationship between the two phenomena by combining both types of mobility (residential and occupational). This would eventually be achieved by Daniel Courgeau, using methods that included conducting a retrospective survey with a view to analysing respondents' mobility event histories.

2.1.1.2 The *Triple Biographie*: *biographie familiale, professionnelle et migratoire* Survey

In 1981, the first life-course survey of 4602 individuals, born between 1911 and 1935 and representative of the French population of these birth cohorts, was conducted by INED. The survey questionnaire recorded the matrimonial history of the respondent and his or her life partner, their birth history, information regarding their children and parents, all periods of employment and economic inactivity, and details of each dwelling inhabited (Courgeau 1984).

The objectives of this survey – called the *Biographie familiale, professionnelle et migratoire* (Family, work and migration event histories) survey, also known as *Enquête 3B* (3B Survey) – were altogether compatible with urban research and the study of residential mobility, while at the same time extending beyond these fields. This survey sought to push the boundaries of conventional demographic analysis by no longer concentrating on specific events (deaths, marriages, births, migration) and instead focusing on individual trajectories considered as a complex process. The analysis of life-event histories would therefore take account of the duration and sequence in time and space of individual trajectories within their social frameworks. This involved analysing the way in which a family-related, occupational or other event changes the probability of other life events occurring, depending on the environment in which it takes place (urban or rural, for example). Among other things, this survey sought to assess the influence that marriage could have on migration to metropolitan areas (Courgeau 1987) or on decisions to leave the farming world (Courgeau and Lelièvre 1986). The result was therefore an analysis of interactions between demographic phenomena – including rural-to-urban migration, marriage and divorce, the birth of children, and individuals' occupational mobility – that also took account of social origins and full life histories. The underlying hypothesis was that these behaviours changed over individuals' lifetimes according to successive personal experiences and acquired knowledge. It was therefore a question of taking into consideration the dynamic heterogeneity within the populations concerned in an analysis that was no longer deterministic but, in principle, probabilistic, and of proposing an alternative to a causal approach.

Previous studies had analysed forms of residential mobility induced by changes in family make-up (Bastide and Girard 1974), with the hypothesis that any modifications in family composition that made the current dwelling unsuitable would lead to migration. *Enquête 3B*, by contrast, considered the interactions between mobility and family-related or occupational changes without presuming that one process had a greater or lesser influence over the other, giving rise to original analyses. This made it possible to further explore migration due to marriage, which had long been studied on the sole basis of extracts from registers of births, deaths and marriages (Courgeau and Lelièvre 1986; Bonvalet and Lelièvre 1991a). Marriage is a time of considerable mobility, when spouses often move into a shared home, but it also marks the start of a period of great residential stability. Depending on marital status, occupation and other personal characteristics that change over an individual's lifetime, different mobility patterns can be identified: high levels of mobility among young people before marriage, especially during higher education and prior to finding a stable job, precede a period of relative stability that is amplified by the transition to home-ownership, among other factors (Courgeau 1985). Moreover, when these interactions are examined, gendered effects also came to light, underlining the disparity between the male and female marriage markets (Courgeau and Lelièvre 1986). And if migration is considered within the framework of the urbanization process and in interaction with fertility, it becomes clear that highly specific behaviours are in operation: specific migrant couples with particularly low fertility choose to move to highly urbanized areas where fertility is below average while, in contrast, fertility rises among those who leave these areas (Courgeau 1984).

This approach assumed that the behaviour of individuals was more adequately modelled as a complex stochastic process. It was then possible to develop a methodology to analyse the operation of different processes in time and space. It was here that the distinction between urban and rural spaces and the changes in behaviour linked to migration from one place to another came into play. This distinction made it possible to explore the data from this survey, which traced and located every key moment of respondents' trajectories.

2.1.1.3 The *Peuplement et dépeuplement de Paris* Survey

The *Peuplement et dépeuplement de Paris* survey, while continuing to address the question developed by Guy Pourcher in his work on population growth in Paris (Pourcher 1963, 1966), had the more specific objective of studying Parisians' housing conditions throughout their lives. It was inspired to a large extent by *Enquête 3B*, but placed the emphasis on the relationship between residential and family trajectories, and on the links between the family and housing. This shift in the framing of the question was quite deliberate: at the start of the 1980s, territorial planning and development issues were less present and the Île-de-France region, with its unappealing living conditions, was becoming less attractive. At the same time, the question of housing was re-emerging, as the existing housing stock was proving insufficient in the face of changing family structures. The tighter focus on housing also corresponded to the phenomenon of rising property ownership during the second half of the twentieth century. This resulted in the hypothesis that residential mobility was partly driven by the desire to become a homeowner ever earlier in the cycle of family life. Indeed, one of the objectives of the survey was to study the acquisition of real estate over respondents' lifetimes.

The survey, conducted in 1986 among 1987 individuals born between 1926 and 1935 and living in the Paris region, included a retrospective section that recorded the conditions of migrants' arrival in Paris, together with a description of all dwellings occupied for more than a year and details of all the people who lived in each of these dwellings. The second part of the questionnaire concerned the working careers of respondents and their life partners, their family origins and the current place of residence of their parents, brothers and sisters, and adult children.[5]

One of the advantages of this survey was that it provided a long-term view and understanding of the issue of housing, unlike analyses conducted on the basis of census data or data from INSEE's *Logement* (Housing) surveys. It was possible to follow a whole birth cohort over time and thus understand the urban changes that had affected the Paris region during the period. Furthermore, comparisons with *Enquête 3B* (Lelièvre 1990), which covered the same birth cohorts (from 1926 to 1935), gave another dimension to research in the field, as it was possible to conduct detailed analyses of the residential and geographical trajectories of an entire group of cohorts and study Parisian filter effects – for the Paris region does indeed "select" its inhabitants: not everyone "goes up" to Paris. The capital is not just a place where people live and start a family, but also a place that people leave in favour of the provinces. A filtering phenomenon was thus at work here, in that Paris attracted a particular population and bade farewell to a second population that was different

[5] It was therefore possible to compare the results of the *Peuplement et dépeuplement de Paris* survey with those of *Enquête 3B* (Bonvalet 1987).

from the first in terms of age, marital status and social category (Bonvalet and Lelièvre 1991b).

A joint analysis of these two INED surveys led to the production of an initial summary of residential trends for these cohorts (Bonvalet and Lelièvre 1989). Their housing trajectories began at a difficult time, in the middle of a housing crisis, before diversifying in response to family-related and occupational events. But this was also a time marked by the massive construction of social housing and easier access to home-ownership following the introduction of homebuyers' loans from the 1950s. The most common residential trajectory for Parisians was to rent and then, for a third of respondents, to buy their own home. However, alongside this "typical trajectory" were also more varied residential histories, including returns to renting after home-ownership (10 %). And while fewer Parisians owned their primary residence in 1986 than the national average for their birth cohort, they were more likely to possess a second home (Lelièvre and Bonvalet 1994).

With regard to geographical trajectories, the analysis of event histories showed how the spatial distribution of a given cohort changed over time. At age 25, some 41 % of respondents residing in Île-de-France lived in the city of Paris,[6] but the proportion was just 25 % at age 50. This development was largely due to the phenomenon of peri-urbanization that appeared from the 1970s onwards, and the attendant possibility of owning a house, as Martine Berger clearly showed in her work on peri-urban dwellers in the Paris region (Berger 2004).

If residential trajectories are complex, it is partly because choices of housing and location cannot be explained by rational, economic factors such as income level, social class or place of work. Other factors are involved, such as the family history and origins of respondents and their life partners. In the *Peuplement et dépeuplement de Paris* survey, the influence of kinship networks and the surprising spatial proximity of members of the same family was clear to see.

These results, which confirmed and perpetuated those obtained by Guy Pourcher, subsequently awakened interest in surveys on sociability networks and kinship, with the aim of gaining a better understanding of the links between family and housing, and between the entourage and residential territory.

Aside from considerations regarding the location of relatives, these explorations were primarily designed to identify networks of interpersonal relationships, based on the assumption that migratory choices are not just individual choices, but also depend on the characteristics of each individual's social network. This altogether recent link established between mobility studies and studies of sociability networks shows the extent to which these two sets of surveys – concerning mobility and residential trajectories on the one hand, and the family and networks on the other – are complementary.

[6] Translator's note: the city of Paris is just one of the eight *départements* (administrative divisions roughly equivalent to English counties or Italian provinces) that make up the Paris region (Île-de-France). In 2011, the city of Paris represented around 19 % of the population of Île-de-France, and 0.9 % of the total area of the region.

2.1.2 The Legacy of Surveys on the Family and Networks

From 1945 to 1974, INED's work on the family focused essentially on the study of fertility and marriage, with the family increasingly being restricted to couples with children. This vision of the family unit was consistent with the theory developed in the 1930s by the American sociologist Talcott Parsons, which held that the traditional family had become isolated from its kinship network, and that part of its functions had in effect been taken over by schools, the state and employers. According to Parsons, the family had changed with industrialization, and roles within the parental couple had become more specialized, with men responsible for providing the household's resources and women in charge of household tasks. The nuclear family was independent from a residential and financial perspective, and ties with ancestors and collateral relatives were greatly diminished. In this regard, Parsons' theory can be traced straight back to Tocqueville, for whom the weakening of intergenerational relationships characterized the family in America, and in particular the decline of lineage: "the family no longer enters the mind except as something vague, indeterminate and uncertain" (de Tocqueville 1835).[7]

Parsons' theory sparked much controversy and spawned a series of studies and surveys from the late 1950s onwards. Very quickly, American sociologists would refute his theory and show that the nuclear family had maintained ties with their families of origin. Curiously, in Europe, it was the urban sociologists Michael Young and Peter Willmott (1957) who, in studying working-class districts of London in 1957, would rediscover the strength of family ties, especially the mother-daughter relationship. This is also what Chombart de Lauwe (1956) observed in analysing the Parisian social space.

In France, however, and at INED in particular, research continued to focus on the nuclear family. This can be explained by the success of this model, "which essentially made it pointless to study relationships between parents and married children" (Roussel 1976), as well as by the concerns of the post-war era and the two decades that followed. The aim was above all to monitor changes in the birth rate and to try to understand the consequences of these changes, as the baby boom had surprised demographers by its magnitude and duration. Surveys initially attempted to determine the level of public information, opinions and attitudes towards issues relating to the (nuclear) family and population. Over time, though, questions evolved to gauge views on themes such as the influence of family allowances on fertility and the standard of living of large families, later moving on to topics such as contraception and falling birth rates (Girard and Zucker 1968); by 1974, they were addressing issues such as sexual relations between young people and the timing of births (Bastide and Girard 1975). As Louis Roussel noted in 1970, however, two new factors would come to the fore and weigh in favour of studying solidarity networks: youth protests on the one hand, visible since the events of May 1968 and liable to

[7] Cited by Cicchelli-Pugeault and Cicchelli 1998, p. 42.

challenge the transmission of traditional values; and increasing life expectancy on the other, which was changing intergenerational relationships (Roussel 1976).

From 1974, INED began to undertake work on kinship networks that formed part of a current of research on forms of interrelationship between family groups and kinship. In the United States, one of the principal proponents of this research, Marvin Sussman, refuted Parsons' theory from the late 1950s onwards by highlighting the close ties that existed between parents and married children (for childcare, holidays, financial assistance, etc.) (Sussman 1959; Sussman and Burchinal 1962). Litwak would later confirm the existence of these ties despite geographical and occupational distance between members of the same family, proposing to rename the family group "the modified extended family" (Litwak 1985). In this way, he highlighted the importance of exchanges between several nuclear families, a sort of "egalitarian coalition (…) that [had] nothing to do with the traditional extended family" (Déchaux 2003, p. 58). Meanwhile, in Europe, Parsons' concept of the family was heavily undermined in the UK by Elizabeth Bott's research on kinship and neighbourly relations in London, and by Michael Young and Peter Willmott, who revealed the importance of kinship networks in a working-class district of London. Other studies by Jean Rémy in Belgium and Philippe Garigue in Canada would also confirm the persistence of intergenerational solidarity in urban and industrial societies (Rémy 1967; Garigue 1956).

If, as Andrée Michel wrote in 1970, "the sociology of the family in the United States [was] far in advance of anything being done in European countries, particularly French-speaking ones", researchers in France made up for lost time from the mid-1970s onwards, producing studies on the themes of the extended family and kinship networks (Michel 1970a). Of course, as early as 1955, Andrée Michel was undertaking original research on parental relationships within manual-worker households (Michel 1955, 1970b), followed, from 1967 onwards, by Agnès Pitrou, who "would call into question the theory of the isolation of urban households with respect to their families of origin". Agnès Pitrou's research, based on a 1972 survey conducted by CRÉDOC (French Research Centre for the Study and Observation of Living Conditions) and CNAF (French National Family Allowance Fund) among 1744 households, was a pioneering study, and her book *Vivre sans famille*? (Living without a family?) quickly became a reference (Pitrou 1978). The surveys on the family network conducted by Louis Roussel in 1974 and Catherine Gokalp in 1976 marked a pivotal moment in the development of surveys on mutual assistance in France, and as such are the "ancestors" of the *Proches et Parents* survey, and thus also of the *Biographies et entourage* survey.

Before going any further, we must emphasize an important point concerning the legacy of surveys on the family. Unlike mobility surveys, all surveys on family networks adopted a cross-sectional approach. The aim of this approach was to take a snapshot in time of the family in order to measure the extent to which support was provided and favours traded among its members, not to reconstruct the family history with a view to interpreting and understanding the snapshot. The latter is, however, one of the objectives of the *Biographies et entourage* survey.

2.1.2.1 The *La famille après le mariage des enfants. Étude des relations entre générations* Survey

In the context of the 1970s, this survey initiated by Louis Roussel and Odile Bourguignon, titled *La famille après le mariage des enfants. Étude des relations entre générations* (The family after the children have married. A study of intergenerational relationships),[8] was designed to fill a research gap in the field of the sociology of the family: "The convergence of results from foreign studies was an invitation to undertake empirical exploratory research covering the entire French population" (Roussel 1976, p. 2). Like works conducted in the United States, the United Kingdom, Austria and Belgium, it was clearly intended to demolish Parsons' concept of the nuclear family. "The first goal was to challenge, as far as contemporary French society was concerned, the idea of a disconnection between the nuclear family household and the households of the two families of origin. First of all, we needed to know whether interactions between generations were frequent or rare, spontaneous or formal. It was also important to understand the true nature of these interactions: were they simply relics of an outdated form of solidarity, or valuable exchanges that were still relevant?" (Roussel 1976, p. 2).

In France, this survey was innovative not only in terms of the theme it addressed – it was the first French survey to focus on the non-isolation of the nuclear family – but also in terms of the methods it used. Louis Roussel, aware of the difficulties inherent in understanding the study of kinship, proceeded with caution, initially conducting 42 semi-structured interviews, the intended purpose of which was to garner concrete examples of trends and to prepare a questionnaire for a quantitative survey. "It was therefore essential, after the initial qualitative approach, to develop an extensible survey that would provide more representative results. Only then would it become possible to say whether a given model for the transmission of property or a given type of service rendered by parents was exceptional or, on the contrary, habitual" (Roussel 1976, p. 4).

In 1974, 2542 individuals were interviewed, comprising 1260 married children under the age of 45 with at least one living parent and 1282 parents aged under 80 with at least one married child. The questionnaire was designed to identify the level of geographical proximity between parents and married children, the level of support provided (especially around the time of the children's marriage), the frequency of visits from married children (with or without their spouses), and to obtain information on a certain number of practices (e.g. premarital cohabitation, engagement) and opinions regarding norms for mutual support and inheritance.

The survey results confirmed the existence of a high level of solidarity between the parents' and children's generations. While it is true that the children were, as Parsons pointed out, independent from a financial and residential standpoint, this independence was not accompanied by a disconnection between generations. More than half of married children (53 %) lived within 20 km of their parents, rising to

[8] *La famille après le mariage des enfants. Étude des relations entre générations* survey was conducted in 1974 by INED.

three quarters when in-laws were included. Where children lived in the same municipality, 75 % of them visited their parents at least once a week (55 % if they lived in a different municipality less than 20 km away), 15 % of children had received help from parents in finding a job, and 10 % had been assisted financially. However, this ongoing solidarity masks certain changes in the nature of family ties. "One married male respondent said that family is where the heart is [...] [T]his would appear to be the new foundation for intergenerational solidarity" (Roussel 1976, p. 243), with feelings now playing a more important role than norms and tradition. The semi-structured interviews complemented the quantitative approach by going beyond the description of phenomena alone and allowing an analysis of intergenerational relationships that revealed a more complex reality made up of compromise, interplay between distance and proximity, and gifts and counter-gifts on the part of both the parents and the married children.

While Louis Roussel's survey did indeed achieve its objective of calling into question the isolation of the nuclear family in French society, it nevertheless had certain limitations – focusing, for example, solely on relationships between parents and married children, whereas the family also includes brothers and sisters, aunts and uncles, nephews and nieces, who together form an individual's family environment. This particular shortcoming would be remedied 2 years later, in 1976, by a survey focusing on family networks.

2.1.2.2 The *Réseau familial* Survey

Catherine Villeneuve-Gokalp's survey, *Le réseau familial* (The family network), conducted shortly after *La famille après le mariage des enfants*, picked up where Louis Roussel left off by addressing issues of residential and social proximity, assistance, interaction and meetings, but in a broader framework that covered the whole extended family. For the first time in France, the size and composition of kinship and family networks would be studied. According to François Héran, Catherine Villeneuve-Gokalp's survey "was the first of its kind. To my knowledge, nothing like it had been carried out before in France. In English-speaking research, such studies were extremely rare and based on non-representative samples of no more than 800 individuals" (Héran 1982, p. 51).

This national survey, conducted in 1976 among 2075 individuals aged 45–64, had two objectives:

- to quantify kinship – the aim was to measure the size of the family group and study its composition, from grandparents to grandchildren, including the collateral relatives of both spouses;
- to analyse the cohesion of the family group by considering the geographical proximity of relatives, the frequency with which they met, and the level of social proximity (based on the occupations of the spouses in each generation); this follows on from studies by Louis Roussel, in particular his 1974 survey *La famille*

après le mariage des enfants, and by Alain Girard, on individuals' choice of spouse (Girard 1974).[9]

In this survey, each respondent was asked to describe, as in a census, their ascendants, descendants and siblings, as well as those of his or her life partner. The survey covered five generations in all, from the respondent's grandparents to the respondent's grandchildren. This family group included 23 people on average and varied little according to the age of the respondent, as the children and grandchildren replaced the grandparents and parents over time.

The *Réseau familial* survey made it possible to analyse the geographical dispersion of the family and highlighted both the extreme proximity of parents' and children's places of residence (63 % of respondents lived within 20 km of their parents) and the intensity of their relationships: 90 % of parents who lived in the same municipality as their daughter saw her at least once a week. While the ties between parents and children, as previously highlighted by Louis Roussel, remained very strong, the same was not true for siblings, who tended to become more emotionally and geographically distant over the years: nearly three in five respondents lived more than 20 km away from their siblings, and only 63 % of those who lived in the same municipality as a sibling saw this sibling every week.

Finally, several secondary uses have also been made of the *Réseau familial* survey. The wealth of data, in particular concerning the occupations of parents and siblings, has made it possible to explore previously little-known domains, such as the transmission of self-employed status from parents to children and the differential social mobility of brothers compared with sisters (Zarca 1993a, b).

2.1.2.3 The *Proches et parents* Survey

The *Proches et parents* survey, which followed on directly from previous surveys conducted by INED in 1970s (Roussel 1976; Gokalp 1978), continued the exploration of the family and elective ties, incorporating acquired knowledge from the *Peuplement et dépeuplement de Paris* survey (Bonvalet 1987) and INSEE and INED's *Contact* survey (Héran 1987), which underlined the role and the social utility of kinship. In *Proches et parents*, the household was finally brought out of the isolation in which it had been considered by studies on the family since the 1950s. With rising unemployment, a difficult housing situation for young people, and increasing numbers of older people, the family had once again found its place in society (Segalen 2006; Bonvalet and Gotman 1993). In addition to co-residence, the role of parents was highlighted on numerous levels, ranging from mutual support to sociability. For this reason, there was a need in the late 1980s for an updated survey on the family network, as the family had undergone significant changes. With the

[9]At this time, Agnès Pitrou was also undertaking innovative research on family solidarity; she made a distinction between two types of support within the family: "subsistence" support and "promotional" support.

increase in divorce and the rise of formerly marginal family configurations (non-marital cohabitation, single-parent families, stepfamilies), the family had become more complex and its boundaries more blurred. Moreover, these changes justified the extension of the survey to interpersonal relationships outside the family. Catherine Villeneuve-Gokalp's survey had illustrated the many potential applications of the approach, but was limited to family configurations, described in terms of kinship. While this approach led to the production of an initial static geography of the family, it told us nothing about the dynamics at play. What were the most important aspects of these family relationships? What did individuals like and dislike about these relationships? In what ways did family members interact? Where did the boundary lie between this particular "constellation" and other sets of relationships (Bonvalet et al. 2007)?

The *Proches et parents* survey, conducted by INED in 1990 among 1946 individuals representative of the adult French population aged 18 and over, had three goals: to increase knowledge of the extended family; to explore the network of affinities; and to study the social uses of family and friendship networks. Questions concerning mutual support focused on the integrating role of the family with regard to employment and housing. Information was also collected on assistance received and given on a regular basis (childcare, help with household tasks, care for the elderly) and during hard times (financial problems, divorce, unemployment, health problems). For each type of assistance, the receivers and givers were identified. The survey was complemented by around 100 unstructured interviews on the subject of residential and family history.[10] The aim was to build upon the relational configurations that emerged from the quantitative survey and the analysis of interviews in order to identify patterns of trajectories and family and residential profiles that were significant with respect to research questions on the household, the family and housing. The cross-matching of quantitative and qualitative data shed light on the role that family plays as an intermediary between the individual and society by encouraging the integration of young people and avoiding the marginalization of the oldest and most vulnerable individuals. Of course, it must be remembered that in addition to providing support, families can also be a source of inequalities, problems and handicaps.

The results of the *Proches et parents* survey once again confirmed the persistence of kinship relations previously demonstrated by numerous studies on intergenerational solidarity, both in France (Pitrou 1978; Segalen 1981; Attias-Donfut 1995; Crenner 1998) and abroad (Dandurand and Ouellette 1992; Coenen-Huther et al. 1994; Bengtson and Roberts 1991). Two thirds of respondents had contact at least once a week with a member of their family, half lived in the same municipality as at least one of their parents, and three quarters said they were close to their mother (Bonvalet et al. 2007). In the vast, vast majority of families, exchanges of assistance and favours took place (Ortalda 2001).

[10]These interviews were conducted and analysed as part of a research programme coordinated by the SRAI (*Statuts résidentiels : approche intergénérationnelle* [Residential statuses: intergenerational approach]) working group (Bonvalet et al. 2007).

While the extended family continues to exist in urban society, despite the rise of individualism, the ties that adult children maintain with their parents are highly variable. Some become more distant over time, while others maintain very close relationships with their families of origin. Just as no single household type exists, neither is there one single type of extended family. Statistical analysis has identified several different forms of kinship. The family entourage – defined using indicators for affinity, frequency of contact and mutual assistance – corresponds to a reality that challenges the hypothesis of a general trends towards withdrawal into the domestic sphere: 30 % of respondents belong to a local family entourage, which means that (a) they live in the same municipality as at least one of their parents, to whom they say they are close, (b) they have contact with this person at least once a week, and (c) they exchange favours and assistance with this person; and 17 % belong to a dispersed family entourage, meaning they maintain this kind of strong relationship but do not live nearby. In total, nearly half of all respondents had kinship ties that operated according to the local family entourage model (Bonvalet 2003).

Women tend to organize their kinship relations in this fashion more than men, and thus appear to be the main builders of family ties and exchanges (Hammer et al. 2001). Although differences exist according to social background (professionals seem slightly less oriented towards the local family entourage than manual workers, for instance), family history and residential history are decisive factors. To summarize, the local family entourage is more the product of the experiences of several generations and lineages than the result of some sort of social or demographic determinism.

The interviews helped to refine this theory by seeking to understand the processes that organize these configurations of family life. Several types of process coexist: some correspond to a "home-making" approach – by reproducing the family model, by adopting the in-laws or, when there is no contact with the two families of origin, by initiating this mode of operation with adult children – while others, by contrast, do not correspond to a real choice. In this case, the local family entourage tends to be the result of an economic or a financial constraint instead. In fact, the local family entourage appears to be both a way of living as a family that respects the independence of each individual and couple – we might even suggest that it is precisely because the family entourage exists that a degree of individual autonomy is possible (Attias-Donfut et al. 2002)[11] – and a means of adapting the complex family to urban society; some respondents favour a lifestyle governed by the interests of the family group, while others did not really choose this way of family life and have to deal with the associated constraints.

These analyses reflect the situations for respondents at the time of the survey and at the time of the interview. Over a lifetime, the same individual may function as part of the local family entourage at certain times and, depending on family or occupational circumstances, as part of the dispersed family entourage at others. This dual behaviour may be initiated by parents – for example, when children move out

[11] For Claudine Attias-Donfut, Nicole Lapierre and Martine Segalen, kinship and individualism are not incompatible, but rather are complementary, even compensatory.

of the family home to a new residence in the local area – or later on by children if they set up home in the same municipality, or even move back in with their parents.

All three surveys – *La famille après le mariage des enfants*, *Réseau familial*, and *Proches et parents* – represented real breakthroughs in research on kinship in their time. Furthermore, together with other cross-sectional surveys conducted by INSEE on kinship networks (Crenner 1998, 1999) and CNAV (the French national pension fund) on intergenerational solidarity (Attias-Donfut 1995), they helped French research to catch up with its English-language counterparts – a fact which Peter Willmott pointed out in January 2000 in his preface to the English edition of the work *La famille et ses proches*, titled *Family Kinship and Place in France*.[12] However, there remained the issue of historical depth, vital for understanding these snapshots in time. Resolving this issue was a key objective of the *Biographies et entourage* survey.

2.1.3 *The* Biographies et entourage *Survey*

Taking account of previous surveys involved a certain amount of selection – deciding what to keep and what to discard – and, as with any legacy, a degree of re-appropriation, finding the right positioning in order to overcome identified limitations and achieve objectives that not only incorporate goals from previous operations, but also present new challenges. Indeed, while some surveys serve to update knowledge, reiterating previous observations, others, like *Biographies et entourage*, explicitly take on both thematic and methodological challenges. This new operation, announced in the "prospects" section of *Biographies d'enquêtes*, published by GRAB (*Groupe de réflexion sur l'approche biographique* – [Working group on event-history approach]), was to follow on methodologically from other life event-history surveys via two objectives in particular: "to introduce the many different places with which an individual has contact [...] and to move from studying individual life-event histories to studying those of a group of individuals". This meant identifying the dynamics of spatial and relational contexts throughout individuals' trajectories, which in turn required careful consideration of how to achieve a "truly quantitative calibration capable of homogenizing narratives whose level of precision varies according to the combined temporal and relational proximity of the individuals that make up the entourage" (GRAB 1999, p. 339).

[12] Peter Willmott wrote in 2000: "I was disappointed when I visited Paris in the late 1960s seeking collaborators for a comparative cross-national study of the extended family. In contrast to their British counterparts, who have been studying kinship from the mid-1950s on, French social researchers then showed little interest in the family apart from its nuclear form. After the mid-1970s, however, a number of studies were undertaken by French researchers, including some at INED. The research on which this book is based comes from the same stable. It shows that the British have now been overtaken" (preface to *Family Kinship and Place in France*, London, Southern Universities Press/INED 2007).

2.1.3.1 Accommodating Legacy Features

As detailed above, two series of surveys have converged and directly contributed to the design of the *Biographies et entourage* survey and to the development of the concept of the entourage. Moreover, the researchers responsible for these legacy surveys (including Daniel Courgeau and Catherine Bonvalet) were involved in both sets of surveys – those related to mobility and residential trajectories, and those related to the family and relationship networks. The *Biographies et entourage* survey has benefited from this dual heritage and, as with any legacy, certain elements from past surveys have been retained and certain innovations have been introduced.

In particular, data from the two most recent surveys in each series – *Peuplement et dépeuplement de Paris* (1986) and *Proches et parents* (1990) – have contributed directly to *Biographies et entourage* by "testing" the feasibility of collecting dynamic information across a network of individuals, and by confirming the utility of studying all the co-residents of an individual throughout his or her life (Bonvalet and Lelièvre 1995b; Lelièvre et al. 1997).

From a longitudinal perspective, the notions of household or family do not correspond to an operational entity. The procedure for "monitoring" a complex group over time can be built around the respondent – for example, the data from the *Peuplement et dépeuplement de Paris* survey identified the composition of an individual's successive co-residence situations, whether in the same dwelling or not. This solution takes account of entourage members who move closer to, or further away from, the respondent, regardless of location. For example, a respondent may move home with his or her life partner (i.e. several dwellings but one continuous co-residence), or may no longer live with his or her children, who have left to settle elsewhere (i.e. one dwelling but with changes in the make-up of the household). From this observation, two principles for quantitative data collection can be determined: first, it is necessary to have a definition that identifies the group uniquely over time, regardless of its spatial location; and second, monitoring of this kind must be centred on a person, not a place. Indeed, the cross-sectional identification on which the definition of the household is founded – the dwelling – loses all legitimacy in a longitudinal analysis, as data collection cannot focus on the changing occupants of a given dwelling over time. Similarly, the concept of the household, whose definition is based on a unity of place, would seem to be unsuitable for taking account of the history of the family group.

From an event-history perspective, each individual trajectory must be considered within its context. While households typically change throughout an individual's life, relationships – especially family relationships – tend to last, regardless of whether the people in question are also co-residents at a given point in time. To account for this reality, we proposed using the concept of the "entourage" that surrounds an individual and incorporates the realms of both the household and the family, as it includes the domestic group as well as the key figures in the family network and the inner circle of friends. This raises the question of how to identify these key people. Individuals can designate themselves, as in the *Proches et parents* survey; or, as outlined above, we can also systematically include parents, children, current life partners, and former life partners (only when there are children) on the basis of these reported data.

To assess the feasibility of reconstructing the trajectory of each respondent's entourage, we simulated such a trajectory using data from the *Proches et parents* survey conducted by INED in 1990. An article presenting the initial results of the survey (Bonvalet et al. 1993) revealed that the number of relatives (ascendants, descendants and collateral relatives) for respondents living with a partner was around 40 in total, while the maximum figure for single respondents stood at 26 – in both cases, extensive groups that would be difficult to monitor. By contrast, choosing to monitor an elective family group within the kinship network, i.e. considering only those family members described as close relatives by the respondent, seems more manageable. Even for couples with a family group of around 40 people, only 5.5 relatives, on average, were identified as being close to the respondent, with young couples reporting the largest number (6.3) and single older men reporting the fewest (2.8). This limited number of close relatives makes monitoring the entourage more feasible. As the respondents surveyed were all aged over 18, we then carried out a simulation of the changes likely to take place within their entourage throughout their lifetimes (Lelièvre et al. 1997). This simulation confirmed that it was possible to identify and follow a small group totalling eight people at most.

The *Biographies et entourage* survey has taken inspiration from *Proches et parents* for the composition of the family network, with information collected for each member of the family (marital status, occupational status, social class, etc.), as well as the notion of *proches* (i.e. people close to an individual), be they family members, friends, work colleagues or neighbours.

It has also drawn upon the longitudinal approach to the domestic group used by the *Peuplement et dépeuplement de Paris* survey, collecting data on the composition of all households occupied by the respondent, on all places of kinship and on any secondary residences or other dwellings.

Specifically, the entourage defined for these purposes, combining concepts of household and family, includes the biological and/or adoptive parents of the respondent; any other people who have played a parental role; siblings; all life partners and their parents; the respondent's children and those of his or her life partners; and grandchildren. Added to this core family group are key people who have marked the respondent's life (other family members, friends, colleagues, etc.) and co-residents, i.e. everyone with whom the respondent has lived for at least 1 year (Table 2.1).

From *Triple biographie*, the *Biographies et entourage* survey has borrowed the principle of collecting data for all three trajectories – family, residential and occupational – and has extended it to members of the entourage.

Having established the membership of the entourage and the principles for reconstituting event histories across the lifetimes of each of these individuals, combining family, residential and occupational information, we also decided that, in the context of this quantitative data collection, information should be gathered from a single person, whose entourage is monitored from his or her birth to the date of the survey.

Table 2.1 Entourage members systematically described in the *Biographies et entourage* survey

Ascendants and descendants	Other friends and relatives
Ascendants	Life partners (married or not, cohabiting or not)[a]
Biological parents[a]	Parents of life partners
Adoptive parents[a]	Children of life partners
Mother's or father's partner(s)[a]	All co-residents with whom the respondent has lived for at least 1 year
Other individuals who have played a parental role	Other key individuals mentioned for their positive or negative role
Collateral relatives	
Siblings	
Half-siblings	
Foster siblings	
Descendants	
Respondent's children	
Respondent's grandchildren	

[a]These individuals' trajectories are recorded exactly; other trajectories are recorded in less detail

These event histories for members of the individual's entourage were therefore collected by interviewing a single reference person (the respondent) using a questionnaire that includes a section for recording precise details of the respondent's own trajectory and a section concerning the individual's entourage. All respondents were prompted to identify the key events marking their own histories – family history, residential trajectory and sequence of activities (occupational or otherwise) – as well as aspects of the life-event histories of their ascendants and descendants (from grandparents to grandchildren) and certain details of their marital background (see Table 2.1).

2.1.3.2 Questionnaire Design

In addition to drawing inspiration from 20 years' experience of event-history data collection in different countries (GRAB 1999), the methodology used in this survey was based on a number of trials[13] and pilot operations used to validate the questionnaire design and test the different phases of data collection, from interviewer training to the processing of questionnaires. These tests were conducted between May 1996 (when a number of preliminary interviews were conducted by researchers) and November 1999, and the data collection tools were fine-tuned in response to the results obtained. Below is a list of the operations for which detailed assessments were produced[13]:

[13]The descriptions of the different tests and their outcomes and contributions are detailed in Reports 1, 2 and 3, reproduced on the CD-ROM which is available in *De la famille à l'entourage*, Bonvalet and Lelièvre (2012).

- November 1997: 64 questionnaires administered by 8 interviewers;
- June–July 1998: 120 questionnaires administered by 12 interviewers, with certain interviews being recorded to improve question formulation;
- September–October 1998: qualitative interviews by members of the research team with ten respondents initially surveyed by questionnaire in June–July;
- December 1998: testing of new question order by three interviewers who had participated in the June questionnaires (entourage then respondent's trajectory);
- May 1999: three new interviewers to test the 3-day interviewer training programme, the new event-history calendar, etc.;
- November 1999: 104 questionnaires administered by 12 interviewers; coordination of the whole procedure, from data collection to follow-up and processing.

The final questionnaire and the collection logistics presented below are the product of all these operations.

2.1.4 Presentation of the Questionnaire

The questionnaire for the *Biographies et entourage* survey, reproduced in the Appendix, is based on test cases to show more clearly how the questionnaire form was filled in. We have reproduced two questionnaires: one is the English translation of the original and one is filled in for "fictional" respondents invented using elements taken from several real life-event histories that were collected and subsequently anonymized and altered. This questionnaire, together with other fictional biographies, were used for the training of the 178 interviewers who administered the survey at various times between March 2000 and September 2001, to the point that they became "real" life-event trajectories for the researchers who trained the interviewers. The questionnaire is divided into three main parts, in which the following data are successively collected (see Boxes 2.1 and 2.2):

1. Occupational and family trajectories of members of the respondent's entourage;
2. Residential, occupational and family-related milestone events that took place in each year of the respondent's trajectory;
3. An open summary, given by the respondent, who is asked to divide his or her life into different periods and characterize each period in comparison to the others.

In the first part of the questionnaire, data collection is based essentially on closed and factual questions, whereas the summary, which concludes the interview, provides the respondent's own interpretation of the progression, landmark events and overall tone of his or her life course.

Far from representing a difficulty, the multidimensional nature of the questions (family-related, occupational and residential) makes it easier for respondents to recall different events thanks to the connections and associations between them. To achieve this, interviewers followed a methodology that allowed respondents to reconstruct their past without the need for precise dates – it would have been

Box 2.1. Detailed Structure and Sequencing of the Questionnaire

I. ***Introduction***

"First of all, we're going to identify the different stages of your family history."

II. ***Your entourage***

"Now, together, let's describe the trajectories of the different members of your entourage."

- Parents and other individuals who played a parental role,
- Siblings,
- Life partners (married, cohabiting or otherwise) and their parents,
- The respondent's children and his/her life partners' children,
- Grandchildren,
- Other individuals close to the respondent.

III. ***Dwellings***

"We're now going to date and describe all the different dwellings in which you have lived for at least a year, from your birth to the present day."

(a) Listing of stages in the respondent's residential trajectory and description of dwellings occupied
(b) Composition of households,
(c) Other places frequented by the respondent.

IV. ***Activities***

"Lastly, we'd like to know a bit more about the various activities you have undertaken – in your working career or otherwise – since the age of 14 or the end of your formal education."

V. ***Summaries***

"Now, using the grid that we filled in together, please give us your interpretation of the information it contains."

VI. ***Conclusion***

Income level,
Intention to move home,
The interviewer and the respondent both have a guide to completing the questionnaire titled *Légendes*, which contains details of the order of the interview, the wording of questions and the codes/terms used in the grid.

unrealistic to expect such detailed recall. Instead, respondents were asked to build up a timeline of events in accurate chronological order (i.e. events from different fields correctly located on the timeline relative to each other), as this is an absolutely essential condition for the subsequent analysis. In the *Biographies et entourage*

Box 2.2. Themes Addressed in the Questionnaire

Family trajectories

- Family histories of the respondent and all members of the entourage: unions, cohabitations, nuptiality, fertility and descendants (including adopted children and stepchildren).

Residential mobility

- Chronological list of dwellings occupied since birth and their characteristics (type of housing, size, household amenities, tenure status and holder of this status, etc.),
- List of different places frequented throughout the respondent's life (type of place and location),
- Residential proximity between the respondent and the members of his/her entourage throughout the residential trajectory (same municipality or neighbouring municipality),
- Places of residence of entourage members at the time of the survey with respect to the respondent's location (co-resident, same municipality, different municipality, different *département*),
- Intention to move home.

Composition of all households in which the respondent has lived

- Changes in the size of the households in which the respondent has lived,
- Changes in the structure of the respondent's households.

Occupational mobility

- Chronological list of periods of employment, unemployment and voluntary work for the respondent, the respondent's parents (biological and adoptive) and the respondent's life partners,
- Main occupations and employment profiles (alternation of periods of employment and unemployment) of the other members of the entourage,
- Presence of family members in the same company/workplace as the respondent.

Respondent's interpretation of the different phases of his/her trajectory

- Respondent's division of his/her life into different periods, and his/her characterization of these periods,
- Milestone events (personal, historical, etc.) and key people,
- Assessment of financial well-being throughout his/her trajectory.

questionnaire, we drew upon the accumulated experiences of previous surveys (GRAB 1999) and adopted a matrix-based collection method for gathering details of respondents' trajectories: the Life History Calendar (Axinn et al. 1997). Event-history data relating to the respondent (combining descriptions of events and circumstances from family, residential and occupational trajectories, along with a breakdown proposed by the respondent in the summary) are collected using the same year-by-year grid, and then dated, described and linked via a common calendar. This grid helps to ensure, from the outset, that the diachronic structure of the narrative is recorded as accurately as possible.

As information on the trajectories of entourage members is collected via a single reference person, the narratives recorded will generally be less accurate than the information provided by respondents about their own trajectories. Previous research (Poulain et al. 1991) has shown the extent to which this testimony can vary according to the nature of the events remembered, the sex of respondents, their age, etc. The aim here is therefore to give consistency to a narrative whose accuracy varies according to the combined temporal and relational proximity of the individuals that make up the entourage. For example, the tests carried out before the full-scale data-collection phase showed that parents' trajectories were recalled much more accurately by respondents than the trajectories of siblings and children. As the quantitative collection of interviews of this kind requires considerable efforts in terms of "fitting" uncertain material, the collection methods used here were adjusted according to the expected "accuracy" of the respondent's narrative (different versions of the data-collection grid and various question orders and wordings were tested during the various steps of this fitting process).

In sum, the data collection method for *Biographies et entourage* has been designed to facilitate the recollection of information by the respondent while adapting to the variable precision of the information collected.

More specifically, the pilot operations for administering and processing the questionnaires made it possible to optimize the questioning procedure and showed, in particular, that it was better to start by recording the trajectories of the entourage, before recording the respondent's personal history. This order provides an initial family framework that facilitates the identification and description process for both the interviewer and the respondent. Moreover, it proved more efficient to gather the most difficult information – that is, information relating to third parties – early in the interview and finish with the respondent's own life (Lelièvre and Vivier 2001).

The core section of the questionnaire – the data-collection grid for the respondent's trajectories – included a flap system that made it possible to view family-related events (marked in the "Family" column), residential phases and occupational phases simultaneously. This arrangement respected the processes involved in retrieving memories, which are built on connections and associations between the different events and circumstances in each field of life events. The respondent's narrative frequently reflected the importance of these types of connections and milestones in memory recall, as evidenced by phrases such as: "I moved to Marseille when I got married". A particular effort was therefore made to ensure that the questionnaire, in its very structure and presentation, focused on practical comparison of the different life-event domains. Both interviewer and respondent had each of these domains constantly in view, enabling them to refer to a previously mentioned event (therefore avoiding the often quite difficult task of dating life events).

In addition, this framework allowed for the easy insertion of forgotten events or steps at any time. For example, military service (which was compulsory in France until the late 1990s) was rarely viewed as a residential step (except in cases where it involved a posting in Algeria or another foreign country); however, it was invariably remembered as an activity. The flexibility of the grid meant that if forgotten initially, it could be simply added as a stage in the respondent's residential history.

The ability to make such connections during the data collection process enabled both the interviewer and the respondent to "find their bearings" within the life-event history, identify any omissions and inconsistencies quickly, and remedy them easily. This framework therefore ensured that the information collected was as homogeneous as possible, while retaining the richness and uniqueness of the narrative.

The observation period covered by the data collection procedure depended on the respondent's family tree, beginning before the respondent's own birth (with a reconstitution of the activities of his/her parents in their youth) and ending with the respondent's grandchildren. The historical depth of observation is therefore greater than the respondent's lifespan in each case, and so, for our sample, extends from the late nineteenth century to the late twentieth century. To achieve this kind of coverage, it was necessary to design a data collection tool that could facilitate memory recall, accommodate very different social realities and adapt to narratives whose accuracy (especially in terms of dates) varies according to the nature of the ties in question and how long ago the various events took place. In particular, the difficulty inherent in recounting the lives of others called for the use of a collection tool that could adapt to the uncertain testimony of a single interviewee. Data collection methods and the list of questions could then be adjusted according to the expected "accuracy" of the respondent's narrative – ranging from precise information concerning family and occupational trajectories for parents and life partners to vague details of family events, main occupations and current places of residence for parents-in-law.

2.1.5 The Survey in the Field

The data collection phase of the survey took place between March 2000 and September 2001. The length of this phase was justified by the essential and highly personalized involvement of researchers with regard to the interviewers and INED's Surveys Department. Logistics in the field were managed by the Surveys Department at INED, assisted by a specially recruited *ad hoc* team.

A total of 178 interviewers were recruited in the Île-de-France region, including interviewers and students selected by INED in response to a published advertisement, interviewers from INSEE's network, and interviewers from the company Action-Hexagone.

Interviewer training, provided by instructors working in pairs, continued throughout the collection process. It was provided by a researcher from the team and a member of INED's Surveys Department, spread over 3 days. The first day was spent showing how the questionnaire works using a case study (see the completed questionnaire in the Appendix). The interviewers then practised administering a questionnaire. The final half-day, devoted to analysing interviewers' data collection experiences, was also an opportunity for a personalized debriefing, in which each interviewer, together with the person responsible for monitoring their work in the field (rereading and checking the consistency of the questionnaires returned), could resolve any problems that might have arisen during the collection process. During the field surveys, regular meetings were organized between interviewers and their monitoring teams.

The interviewers were provided with address files in order to contact respondents once a notification letter had been sent out to them. Once appointments had been made for both the tests and the actual survey, all scheduled interviews were successfully completed.

The information collected was very dense, and therefore had to be codified with special care in order to conserve as much detail as possible. In particular, information concerning occupations and additional remarks (noted in the many different spaces provided for this purpose) was treated separately. The monitoring team carried out these and all associated tasks, from rereading and codification to questionnaire data entry. This team – comprising eight full-time staff members who were all trained in each of these tasks – continued working after data collection had been completed, in order to perform the necessary data auditing. Certain members of this experienced team were also charged with coding the open questions and creating specific variables.

2.1.6 The Survey Sample

2.1.6.1 Birth Cohorts Surveyed

The choice of cohorts to be surveyed was also made with reference to the previous surveys that paved the way for *Biographies et entourage*. The *Peuplement de Paris* survey, for instance, collected data from cohorts born between 1901 and 1911; *Triple biographie* concerned cohorts born between 1911 and 1935; and *Peuplement et dépeuplement de Paris* surveyed residents of Île-de-France born between 1926 and 1935. The respondents in the *Biographies et entourage* survey were all born between 1930 and 1950, thus allowing the analysis of residential and family trajectories for cohorts of Île-de-France residents born between 1900 and 1950.

The individuals surveyed for *Biographies et entourage*, aged between 50 and 70 in 2000, represented pioneering cohorts at a key junctures in their lives:

- at key junctures because, on the one hand, they were frequently called upon to help offspring who were having difficulty entering the employment and housing markets, and, on the other, also had to support elderly parents whose life expectancy had increased significantly, but who were experiencing health problems and a loss of independence;
- pioneers because they had lived through, and participated in, the great transformations of the second half of the twentieth century, marked by the massive entry of women into the labour force, the development of contraception that made it easier for them to reconcile work and family life, and changing family configurations, with growing numbers of single-parent families and stepfamilies;
- last, at the end of the housing crisis of the 1950s, these cohorts were the stakeholders of urban changes affecting the Île-de-France region, with the revitalization of town and city centres and the rise of peri-urbanization; they have thus initiated new urban lifestyles both in urban contexts (gentrification) and in rural areas, with easy access to social housing and ultimately to ownership of a house in the inner or outer suburbs.

The sample (2830 individuals) is large enough to analyse different trends – family-related, occupational and residential – and compare them for each cohort. For example:

- are the baby-boomer cohorts (born between 1946 and 1950) different from the cohorts of the interwar period and the beginning of World War II?
- how have these cohorts initiated new forms of matrimonial behaviour?
- the baby-boomers entering the housing market in the late 1960s and early 1970s, when large high-rise housing estates were being built, were reaching maturity when the Barre-Ornano housing reform law of 1977 came into force, creating personalized housing benefits (*aide personnalisée au logement*, or *APL*, in French); how did their geographical and residential trajectories differ from those of previous generations?

2.1.6.2 Geographical Coverage and Sample Size

The pilot operations that had confirmed the feasibility of the survey had also pointed up the complexity of its data collection requirements and the need for increased involvement of the survey monitoring team. As detailed above, the questionnaire processing chain included frequent exchanges between the questionnaire rereading and coding team and the interviewers, who were the only people authorized to contact respondents again should the need arise. The effort and cost represented by such an operation rapidly raised the issue of the level of geographical coverage that could reasonably be envisaged. With a sample size not expected to exceed 3000, limitations in terms of capability for data collection monitoring and future analysis guided the choice between a dispersed national survey and a denser regional survey; the decision was made to restrict the survey to the Île-de-France region only.

The *Biographies et entourage* survey was subsequently conducted from March 2000 to September 2001.

2.1.6.3 Selecting the Sample Population

Initially, the sample population was to be constituted by directly selecting individuals – on the basis of their age, sex and place of residence – from the sample taken for the National Family survey conducted at the same time as the 1999 French national census; however, this initial sample had to be supplemented by a selection from the census itself.

- the sample is drawn randomly from the sample used for the *Étude de l'histoire familiale* survey (the *Famille* survey) associated with the 1999 census, and from the 1999 census itself;
- for the city of Paris proper, the sample was representative of the sex, age and geographical distribution (by *arrondissement*[14]) of the Parisian population aged 50–70 in 2000;
- for the inner and outer suburbs, municipalities (*communes*) were selected according to Nicole Tabard's nomenclature (Tabard 1993a, b) and a representative sample was then drawn, based on the sex and age distribution of the population concerned;
- each of the five designated post-war new towns in the Île-de-France region (Cergy-Pontoise, Évry, Marne-la-Vallée, Saint-Quentin-en-Yvelines, Sénart) is represented; in fact, the five combined are slightly over-represented in terms of population (11 % instead of 7 %), the objective being to have a minimum of 300 interviews in these areas.

The result was a sample with the following geographical distribution, each regional subset being representative of the area and cohorts surveyed:

City of Paris	585 individuals
Inner suburbs (excluding new towns)	998 individuals
Outer suburbs (excluding new towns)	1263 individuals
New towns	350 individuals

With regard to sex and age composition (Table 2.2), two thirds of respondents were in their 50s, and women were slightly more numerous than men, forming 52 % of the sample.

Consequently, the data gathered by the *Biographies et entourage* survey reveal changes in family structures and the context in which new family configurations (single-parent households, reconstituted families, etc.) have appeared. These data also lend themselves to exploring the ways in which families function, especially in terms of residential practices (dual residence, non rent-paying tenancy, non-

[14] The city of Paris is divided into 20 administrative districts called *arrondissements*.

Table 2.2 Sample composition by sex and age

Age	50–60		61–70		Total (persons)
	N	%	N	%	
Men	869	64.7	474	35.3	1343
Women	976	65.6	511	34.4	1487
Total	1845	65.2	985	34.8	2830

cohabiting couples, etc.). Particular attention has been paid to collecting information on transfers and disruptions – family-related, occupational and residential – across the three generations of individuals covered by this survey. The data collected also provide scope for an analysis of individuals' networks of solidarity and influence and how these networks change throughout their lives.

While building on previous knowledge, the *Biographies et entourage* survey broke new ground in a number of areas, in particular:

- extending the collection of information on family, residential and occupational trajectories to members of the respondent's entourage, including informal situations (early stages of non-cohabiting unions, voluntary activities, alternative places of residence, e.g. boarding schools, barracks);
- identifying and collecting information about figures of elective kinship and the key people in the respondent's entourage;
- taking account of all successive life partners, and of their immediate ascendants and descendants;
- gathering information about places frequented on a regular basis by respondents, and other places of belonging over the course of their lives, including second homes and the circumstances of their acquisition;
- collecting subjective summaries – i.e. recording respondents' "experiences of their own trajectories" and milestone events in their lives, well-being histories together with a financial summary (assessment of their living standards) throughout their life courses.

Additionally, at the time of the survey, the respondents in our sample were at an important stage of their lives, either on the eve of retirement or already retired (possibly before the legal age) with, statistically, many years still ahead of them. As such, this is often a time for potential new beginnings in terms of activities and residential choices – but it is also a time when emotional and family investments may become more diverse or take on a new focus (e.g. on grandchildren or a new life partner). Whatever respondents' plans, they can be considered from the perspective of their trajectories and the trajectories of their entourage.

Appendix

English Translation of the Biographies et entourage *Survey Questionnaire*

Interview start time: |__|__|__|

We are going to build up a picture of your life story and the story of your extended family.
We will start by listing the key dates in your family history.

Q0 What is your first name? .... **Sex:** F 2   M 1

Q1 What is your date of birth? |__|__| *Day* |__|__| *Month*   **19** |__|__| *Year*

Q2 Your place of birth?

Province or country ....

City (*community*) ....

Q3a What is (are) your current nationality?

....

Q3o Has your nationality changed?

No ☐   Yes ☐   Which .... year |__|__|

.... year |__|__|

.... year |__|__|

.... year |__|__|

Q4d What is the highest level/diploma of education you have obtained?

.... None ☐

Q4a Number of schooling years

....

Q5 What is your current marital status?

Single (never married) —— **1**
Married for the first time —— **2**
Separated —— **3**
Divorced or legally separated —— **4**
Remarried —— **5**
Widow/Widower —— **6**

Q6 Do you currently live with someone as a couple (married or unmarried)?

Yes —— **1**
Yes, part time —— **2**
No —— **3**

Q7 How many times have you been married? —— |__|__|

Q8 Excluding your marriage(s), how many times have you been in a couple for <u>more than one year</u>? —— |__|__|

|__|__| **Total number of unions**

Q9 Dates of marriages or unions:

Partner's given name	If married: Marriage	If married: Began living together	If not married: Began living together	If not married: If not living together beginning of relationship	Separation	Divorce	Death	*Family codes to report*
1.	M1	C1	C1	DR1	S1	D1	DCC1	**M1 – M4**
2.	M2	C2	C2	DR2	S2	D2	DCC2	**C1 – C4**
3.	M3	C3	C3	DR3	S3	D3	DCC3	**DR1 – DR4**
4.	M4	C4	C4	DR4	S4	D4	DCC4	**S1 – S4**
								D1 – D4
								DCC1 – DCC4

Q10 Year of birth and (if applicable) death of your parents:

	Given name	Birth	Municipality, province (country)	Death	Notes	
Father :						**DCP**
Mother:						**DCM**

Q11 How many brothers, sisters, half-brothers/sisters do you have?

Sex	Given name	Birth	Death	Notes	
	1.				**NF1, DCF1**
	2.				**NF2, DCF2**
	3.				**NF3, DCF3**
	4.				**NF4, DCF4**
	5.				**NF5, DCF5**
	6.				**NF6, DCF6**
	7.				**NF7, DCF7**
	8.				**NF8, DCF8**
	9.				**NF9, DCF9**
	10.				**NF10, DCF10**
	11.				**NF11, DCF11**
	12.				**NF12, DCF12**
	13.				**NF13, DCF13**
	14.				**NF14, DCF14**
	15.				**NF15, DCF15**

Q13 How many children do you have?

Sex	Given name	Birth	Death	Notes	
	1.				**NE1, DCE1**
	2.				**NE2, DCE2**
	3.				**NE3, DCE3**
	4.				**NE4, DCE4**
	5.				**NE5, DCE5**
	6.				**NE6, DCE6**
	7.				**NE7, DCE7**
	8.				**NE8, DCE8**
	9.				**NE9, DCE9**
	10.				**NE10, DCE10**

YOUR FAMILY

Now let us try to map out the life histories of the members of your extended family

FATHER

Describe the major family events in your father's life	We will now outline the history of your father's activities. What was his occupation when you were born?				
	Precise occupation and periods out of work (*specify interruption for children, illness, unemployment, etc.*)	Statut (1, 2, 3, 4)	Activity of business	Place of work (*municipality, province*)	When? Chronological markers
	First activity PP				*At what age? Up to when?*
	....	....	....	....	....
	....	....	....	....	....
	Next				
	....	....	....	....	....
	....	....	....	....	....
	....	....	....	....	....
Date next events	*At your birth PN*				*Since when?*
You	....	....	....	....	....
....	....	....	....	....	....
....	....	....	....	....	....
....	*Next*				
....	....	....	....	....	....
....	....	....	....	....	....
....	....	....	....	....	....
....	....	....	....	....	....
....	....	....	....	....	....
....	....	....	....	....	....
....	....	....	....	....	....
....	*Last activity DP*				
....	....	....	....	....	....
....	....	....	....	....	....
....	*Retired* ☐	....	....	....	*At what age? When?* ....
....	....	....	....	....	....

- **Did he experience periods of inactivity or interruptions due to war, unemployment, illness, children, return to school, etc?**
  If yes, place them in the chronology.

AP **To summarize: in your opinion, what was his main occupation** (*be specific*) **?**

....

1. Self-employed **2.** Public sector worker (specify) ....

3. Private sector worker **4.** Other (specify) ....

Activity of his business: ....
(*e.g. mechanic: manufacturing, repair*)

HAB **Currently (or prior to his death), does (did) your father live:**

0. With you **100.** In the same or adjacent municipality. Which one: ....

Elsewhere: Municipality, province, country ....

FRE **Currently (or prior to his death), how frequently do (did) you have contact with him?** ....

→ **PROX** **Are (were) you close?** **1.** **2.** **3.** **0.** (does not know)

Where were your paternel grandparents born (region, province or country)

DGPP **Paternel GRANDFATHER?** .... **DGMP** **Paternel GRANDMOTHER?** ....

MOTHER

Describe the major family events in your mother's life	Precise occupation and periods out of work (*specify interruption for children, illness, unemployment, etc.*)	Statut (1, 2, 3, 4)	Activity of business	Place of work (*municipality, province*)	When? Chronological markers
	We will now outline the history of your mother's activities. What was her occupation when you were born?				
	First activity PP				*At what age? Up to when?*
	....	...	....	....	....
	....	...	....	....	....
	Next				
	....	...	....	....	....
	....	...	....	....	....
	....	...	....	....	....
Date next events	*At your birth PN*				*Since when?*
You	....	...	....	....	....
....	....	...	....	....	....
....	....	...	....	....	....
....	*Next*				
....	....	...	....	....	....
....	....	...	....	....	....
....	....	...	....	....	....
....	....	...	....	....	....
....	....	...	....	....	....
....	....	...	....	....	....
....	....	...	....	....	....
....	*Last activity DP*				
....	....	...	....	....	....
....	....	...	....	....	....
....	*Retired* ☐	...	....	....	*At what age? When?* ....
....	....	...	....	....	....

• **Did she experience periods of inactivity or interruptions due to war, unemployment, illness, children, return to school, etc?**
If yes, place them in the chronology.

AP **To summarize: in your opinion, what was her main occupation** (*be specific*) **?**

....

1. Self-employed **2.** Public sector worker (specify) ....

3. Private sector worker **4.** Other (specify) ....

Activity of her business: ....
(*e.g.perfumery: manufacture or commerce*)

HAB **Currently (or prior to her death), does (did) your mother live:**

0. With you **100.** In the same or adjacent municipality. Which one: ....

Elsewhere: Municipality, province, country ....

FRE **Currently (or prior to her death), how frequently do (did) you have contact with her?** ....

→ PROX **Are (were) you close? 1. 2. 3. 0.** (pas connue)

Where were your maternel grandparents born (region, province or country)

DGPP **Maternel GRANDFATHER?** .... DGMP **Maternel GRANDMOTHER?** ....

ADOPTIVE PARENTS OR STEP-FATHER/MOTHER ***(who lived with you)***

Given name: .... **Sex:** F2 M1 **Relationship :** ....

Describe the major family events, in his or her life	**We will now outline the history of his or her activities. What was his or her occupation at the beginning of your relationship?**				
	Precise occupations and periods out of work *(specify interruption for children, illness, unemployment, etc.)*	**Statut** (1, 2, 3, 4)	**Activity of business**	**Place of work** *(municipality, province)*	**When? Chronological markers**
	First activity PP				*At what age? Up to whe?*
	....	....	....	....	....
	....	....	....	....	....
	Next				
	....	....	....	....	....
	....	....	....	....	....
	....	....	....	....	....
DR ⎿⊥⏌ *Date next events*					
....	....	....	....	....	....
....	....	....	....	....	....
....	*Next*				
....	....	....	....	....	....
....	....	....	....	....	....
....	....	....	....	....	....
....	....	....	....	....	....
....	....	....	....	....	....
....	....	....	....	....	....
....	....	....	....	....	....
....	*Last activity DP*				
....	....	....	....	....	....
....	....	....	....	....	....
....	*Retired* ☐	....	....	....	*At what age? When?* ....
....	....	....	....	....	....

- **Did he or she experience periods of inactivity or interruptions due to war, unemployment, illness, children, return to school, etc?** ***If yes, place them in the chronology.***

AP **To summarize: in your opinion, what was his or her main occupation** *(be specific)* **?**

....

1. Self-employed **2.** Public sector worker (specify) ....

3. Private sector worker **4.** Other (specify) ....

Activity of his or her business: ....
(e.g. aviation: plant or transport)

DN **What municipality, province or country was he or she born?** ....

HAB **Currently (or prior to his or her death), does (did) he or she live:**

0. With you **100.** In the same or adjacent municipality. Which one: ....

Elsewhere: Municipality, province, country ....

FRE **Currently (or prior to his or her death), how frequently do (did) you have contact with him or her?** ....

→ **PROX** **Are (were) you close?** **1.** **2.** **3.** **0.** (does not know)

ADOPTIVE PARENTS OR STEP-FATHER/MOTHER ***(who lived with you)***

Given name: .... **Sex:** F2 M1 **Relationship :** ....

Describe the major family events, in his or her life	We will now outline the history of his or her activities. What was his or her occupation at the beginning of your relationship?				
	Precise occupations and periods out of work (*specify interruption for children, illness, unemployment, etc.*)	**Statut** (1, 2, 3, 4)	**Activity of business**	**Place of work** (*municipality, province*)	**When? Chronological markers**
	First activity PP				*At what age? Up to whe?*
	....	....	....	....	....
	....	....	....	....	....
	Next				
	....	....	....	....	....
	....	....	....	....	....
	....	....	....	....	....
DR └─┴─┘ *Date next events*					
....	....	....	....	....	....
....	....	....	....	....	....
....	*Next*				
....	....	....	....	....	....
....	....	....	....	....	....
....	....	....	....	....	....
....	....	....	....	....	....
....	....	....	....	....	....
....	....	....	....	....	....
....	....	....	....	....	....
....	*Last activity DP*				
....	....	....	....	....	....
....	....	....	....	....	....
....	*Retired* ☐	....	....	....	*At what age? When?* ....
....	....	....	....	....	....

• **Did he or she experience periods of inactivity or interruptions due to war, unemployment, illness, children, return to school, etc?** ***If yes, place them in the chronology.***

AP **To summarize: in your opinion, what was his or her main occupation** (*be specific*) **?**

....

1. Self-employed **2.** Public sector worker (specify) ....

3. Private sector worker **4.** Other (specify) ....

Activity of his or her business: ....
(*e.g. aviation: plant or transport*)

DN **What municipality, province or country was he or she born?** ....

HAB **Currently (or prior to his or her death), does (did) he or she live:**

0. With you **100.** In the same or adjacent municipality. Which one: ....

Elsewhere: Municipality, province, country ....

FRE **Currently (or prior to his or her death), how frequently do (did) you have contact with him or her?** ....

→ PROX **Are (were) you close?** **1.** **2.** **3.** **0.** (does not know)

Have there been OTHER PEOPLE who have played a PARENTAL ROLE in your life?

Given name : .... **Sex :** F2 M1 **Relationship:** ....

Describe the major family events in his or her life
(record in chronological order)

Beginning of relationship

Year |__|__|

During what period was his or her influence determinant? (***childhood, adolescence, youth, etc.***)

.... from .... years old to .... years old.

HABp **During this period, did he or she live:**

0. With you **100.** In the same or adjacent municipality. Which one: ....

Elsewhere: Municipality, province, country ....

FREp **How frequent was your contact with this person during this period?** ....

→ **Why was this person important to you? In what way did he or she play a parental role?**

....

....

....

....

....

AP **In your opinion, what was his or her main occupation** (*be specific*) **?**

....

1. Self-employed **2.** Public sector worker (specify) ....

3. Private sector worker **4.** Other (specify) ....

Activity of his or her business: ....
(*e.g. aviation: plant or transport*)

HAB **Currently (or prior to his or her death), does (did) he or she live:**

0. With you **100.** In the same or adjacent municipality. Which one: ....

Elsewhere: Municipality, province, country ....

FRE **Currently (or prior to his or her death), how frequently do (did) you have contact with him or her?** ....

→ **PROX** **Are (were) you close?** **1.** **2.** **3.** **0.** (does not know)

SIBLINGS: Brothers, sisters
half- and step-brothers/sisters, including deceased |__|__|

Occupation profile: A : at work **F :** at home **C :** unemployed
E : studies **M :** illness **R :** retired

Given name : ....

Family events: ⟶

Did you ever live together? **1 Yes.** **2. No**

Currently (or prior to his or her death), does (did) he or she live:

0. With you **100.** In the same or adjacent municipality. Which one: ....

Elsewhere: city, prov., country: ....

Frequency of contact: ....

Are (were) you close? **1.** **2.** **3.** **0.** (does not know)

Main occupation: ....

1. Self-employed **2.** Public sector worker **3.** Private sector worker

Main occupation of partner: ....

1. Self-employed **2.** Public sector worker **3.** Private sector worker

---

Given name : ....

Family events: ⟶

Did you ever live together? **1 Yes.** **2. No**

Currently (or prior to his or her death), does (did) he or she live:

0. With you **100.** In the same or adjacent municipality. Which one: ....

Elsewhere: city, prov., country: ....

Frequency of contact: ....

Are (were) you close? **1.** **2.** **3.** **0.** (does not know)

Main occupation: ....

1. Self-employed **2.** Public sector worker **3.** Private sector worker

Main occupation of partner: ....

1. Self-employed **2.** Public sector worker **3.** Private sector worker

---

Given name : ....

Family events: ⟶

Did you ever live together? **1 Yes.** **2. No**

Currently (or prior to his or her death), does (did) he or she live:

0. With you **100.** In the same or adjacent municipality. Which one: ....

Elsewhere: city, prov., country: ....

Frequency of contact: ....

Are (were) you close? **1.** **2.** **3.** **0.** (does not know)

Main occupation: ....

1. Self-employed **2.** Public sector worker **3.** Private sector worker

Main occupation of partner: ....

1. Self-employed **2.** Public sector worker **3.** Private sector worker

FIRST PARTNER

Given name: .... **Year of birth:** ⌊_ _⌋ **Place of birth** (*city, prov., country*) **:** ....

- **Describe your partner's series of family events (unions, children, etc.).**
  (*circle the union and/or marriage with respondent*)

———————————————————————————————→

- **Highest diploma obtained:** .... None ☐

We will now outline the history of your partner's activities. What was his or her occupation when the relationship began?

Precise occupation and periods out of work (*specify interruption for children, illness, unemployment, etc.*)	Statut (1, 2, 3, 4)	Activity of business	Place of work (*municipality, province*)	When? Chronological markers
First activity PP				*At what age? Up to when?*
....	....	....	....	....
....	....	....	....	....
....	....	....	....	....
Next				
....	....	....	....	....
....	....	....	....	....
....	....	....	....	....
....	....	....	....	....
At the beginning of thr relationship PMC				*Since when?*
If student ↓	....	....	....	....
....	....	....	....	....
....	....	....	....	....
....	....	....	....	....
....	....	....	....	....
....	....	....	....	....
Last activity DP				
....	....	....	....	....
Retired ☐	....	....	....	*At what age? When?* ....
....	....	....	....	....

- **Did your partner experience periods of inactivity or interruptions due to war, unemployment, illness, children, return to school, etc?** ***If yes, place them in the chronology***

AP **To summarize: in your opinion, what is (was) his or her main occupation** (*be specific*) **?**

....

1. Self-employed **2.** Public sector worker (specify) ....

3. Private sector worker **4.** Other (specify) ....

Activity of his or her business: ....
(*e.g. aviation: manufacture or repair*)

- **IF SEPARATED** (part time couple, geographical separation, break up of relationship)

Currently (or before his or her death) did your partner live

100. In the same or adjacent municipality. Which one: ....

Elsewhere: Municipality, province, country..

Currently (or before his or her death), how frequently are (were) you in contact with your partner? ....

SECOND PARTNER

Given name: .... **Year of birth:** |__|__| **Place of birth** (*city, prov., country*) **:** ....

• **Describe your partner's series of family events (unions, children, etc.).**
(*circle the union and/or marriage with respondent*)

• **Highest diploma obtained:** .... None ☐

We will now outline the history of your partner's activities. What was his or her occupation when the relationship began?

Precise occupation and periods out of work (*specify interruption for children, illness, unemployment, etc.*)	Statut (1, 2, 3, 4)	Activity of business	Place of work (*municipality, province*)	When? Chronological markers
First activity PP				*At what age? Up to when?*
....	....	....	....	....
....	....	....	....	....
....	....	....	....	....
Next				
....	....	....	....	....
....	....	....	....	....
....	....	....	....	....
....	....	....	....	....
At the beginning of thr relationship PMC				*Since when?*
If student →	....	....	....	....
....	....	....	....	....
....	....	....	....	....
....	....	....	....	....
....	....	....	....	....
....	....	....	....	....
Last activity DP				
....	....	....	....	....
Retired ☐	....	....	....	*At what age? When?* ....
....	....	....	....	....

• **Did your partner experience periods of inactivity or interruptions due to war, unemployment, illness, children, return to school, etc?** ***If yes, place them in the chronology***

AP **To summarize: in your opinion, what is (was) his or her main occupation** (*be specific*) **?**

....

1. Self-employed **2.** Public sector worker (specify) ....

3. Private sector worker **4.** Other (specify) ....

Activity of his or her business: ....
(*e.g. aviation: manufacture or repair*)

• **IF SEPARATED** (part time couple, geographical separation, break up of relationship)

Currently (or before his or her death) did your partner live

100. In the same or adjacent municipality. Which one: ....

Elsewhere: Municipality, province, country..

Currently (or before his or her death), how frequently are (were) you in contact with your partner? ....

PARTNER'S PARENTS ***Total number*** |__|__|

FATHER-IN-LAW **PARENTS of:** .... **MOTHER-IN-LAW**

Given name : ....
Family events: Partner
Currently (or prior to his death), does (did) he live:
0. With you
100. In the same or adjacent municipality. Which one: ....
Elsewhere: city, prov., country: ....
Frequency of contact: ....
Are (were) you close? **1.** **2.** **3.** **0.** (does not know)
Main occupation: ....
1. Self-employed **2.** Public sector worker **3.** Private sector worker
Activity of business: ....

Given name : ....
Family events: Partner
Currently (or prior to his death), does (did) he live:
0. With you
100. In the same or adjacent municipality. Which one: ....
Elsewhere: city, prov., country: ....
Frequency of contact: ....
Are (were) you close? **1.** **2.** **3.** **0.** (does not know)
Main occupation: ....
1. Self-employed **2.** Public sector worker **3.** Private sector worker
Activity of business: ....

....
....
....
....

FATHER-IN-LAW **PARENTS of:** .... **MOTHER-IN-LAW**

Given name : ....
Family events: Partner
Currently (or prior to his death), does (did) he live:
0. With you
100. In the same or adjacent municipality. Which one: ....
Elsewhere: city, prov., country: ....
Frequency of contact: ....
Are (were) you close? **1.** **2.** **3.** **0.** (does not know)
Main occupation: ....
1. Self-employed **2.** Public sector worker **3.** Private sector worker
Activity of business: ....

Given name : ....
Family events: Partner
Currently (or prior to his death), does (did) he live:
0. With you
100. In the same or adjacent municipality. Which one: ....
Elsewhere: city, prov., country: ....
Frequency of contact: ....
Are (were) you close? **1.** **2.** **3.** **0.** (does not know)
Main occupation: ....
1. Self-employed **2.** Public sector worker **3.** Private sector worker
Activity of business: ....

....
....
....
....

FATHER-IN-LAW **PARENTS of:** .... **MOTHER-IN-LAW**

Given name : ....
Family events: Partner
Currently (or prior to his death), does (did) he live:
0. With you
100. In the same or adjacent municipality. Which one: ....
Elsewhere: city, prov., country: ....
Frequency of contact: ....
Are (were) you close? **1.** **2.** **3.** **0.** (does not know)
Main occupation: ....
1. Self-employed **2.** Public sector worker **3.** Private sector worker
Activity of business: ....

Given name : ....
Family events: Partner
Currently (or prior to his death), does (did) he live:
0. With you
100. In the same or adjacent municipality. Which one: ....
Elsewhere: city, prov., country: ....
Frequency of contact: ....
Are (were) you close? **1.** **2.** **3.** **0.** (does not know)
Main occupation: ....
1. Self-employed **2.** Public sector worker **3.** Private sector worker
Activity of business: ....

....
....
....
....

YOUR CHILDREN *Total* ⌊__⌋

Activity profile: A : at work **F :** at home **C :** unemployed **E :** studies **M :** illness **R :** retired

Given name : ....

If several unions, child of: ....

Family events: →

Currently (or prior to his or her death), does (did) this child live:

0. With you **100.** In the same or adjacent municipality. Which one: ....

Elsewhere: city, prov., country: ....

Frequency of contact: ....

Are (were) you close? 1. 2. 3. 0. (does not know)

Studies in progress: ....

Highest diploma obtained: ....

Main occupation: ....

1. Self-employed **2.** Public sector worker **3.** Private sector worker

Main occupation of partner: ....

1. Self-employed **2.** Public sector worker **3.** Private sector worker

Given name : ....

If several unions, child of: ....

Family events: →

Currently (or prior to his or her death), does (did) this child live:

0. With you **100.** In the same or adjacent municipality. Which one: ....

Elsewhere: city, prov., country: ....

Frequency of contact: ....

Are (were) you close? 1. 2. 3. 0. (does not know)

Studies in progress: ....

Highest diploma obtained: ....

Main occupation: ....

1. Self-employed **2.** Public sector worker **3.** Private sector worker

Main occupation of partner: ....

1. Self-employed **2.** Public sector worker **3.** Private sector worker

Given name : ....

If several unions, child of: ....

Family events: →

Currently (or prior to his or her death), does (did) this child live:

0. With you **100.** In the same or adjacent municipality. Which one: ....

Elsewhere: city, prov., country: ....

Frequency of contact: ....

Are (were) you close? 1. 2. 3. 0. (does not know)

Studies in progress: ....

Highest diploma obtained: ....

Main occupation: ....

1. Self-employed **2.** Public sector worker **3.** Private sector worker

Main occupation of partner: ....

1. Self-employed **2.** Public sector worker **3.** Private sector worker

CHILDREN of your partner(s), from a different union ***Total*** |__|__|

Activity profile: A : at work **F :** at home **C :** unemployed **E :** studies **M :** illness **R :** retired

Given name : .... **Sex :** F2 M1 **Âge** |__|__|
If several partners, child of:........................
Family events: →
Currently (or prior to his or her death), does (did) this child live:
0. With you **100.** In the same or adjacent municipality. Which one: ....
Elsewhere: city, prov., country: ....
Frequency of contact: ....
Are (were) you close? 1. 2. 3. 0. (does not know)
Studies in progress: ....
Highest diploma obtained: ....
Main occupation: ....
1. Self-employed **2.** Public sector worker **3.** Private sector worker
Main occupation: ....
1. Self-employed **2.** Public sector worker **3.** Private sector worker

Given name : .... **Sex :** F2 M1 **Âge** |__|__|
If several partners, child of:........................
Family events: →
Currently (or prior to his or her death), does (did) this child live:
0. With you **100.** In the same or adjacent municipality. Which one: ....
Elsewhere: city, prov., country: ....
Frequency of contact: ....
Are (were) you close? 1. 2. 3. 0. (does not know)
Studies in progress: ....
Highest diploma obtained: ....
Main occupation: ....
1. Self-employed **2.** Public sector worker **3.** Private sector worker
Main occupation: ....
1. Self-employed **2.** Public sector worker **3.** Private sector worker

Given name : .... **Sex :** F2 M1 **Âge** |__|__|
If several partners, child of:........................
Family events: →
Currently (or prior to his or her death), does (did) this child live:
0. With you **100.** In the same or adjacent municipality. Which one: ....
Elsewhere: city, prov., country: ....
Frequency of contact: ....
Are (were) you close? 1. 2. 3. 0. (does not know)
Studies in progress: ....
Highest diploma obtained: ....
Main occupation: ....
1. Self-employed **2.** Public sector worker **3.** Private sector worker
Main occupation: ....
1. Self-employed **2.** Public sector worker **3.** Private sector worker

GRANDCHILDREN

Given name : .... **Sex :** F2 M1 **Age :** |__|__| **or year of birth:** |__|__|__|__|
Child of: ....
Frequency of contact: .... Lives with you
Does this child ever stay into your home without the parents? **1.** Yes **2.** No
How often or on what occasions? ....
....
Are (were) you close? **1.** **2.** **3.** **0.** (does not know) ←

Given name : .... **Sex :** F2 M1 **Age :** |__|__| **or year of birth:** |__|__|__|__|
Child of: ....
Frequency of contact: .... Lives with you
Does this child ever stay into your home without the parents? **1.** Yes **2.** No
How often or on what occasions? ....
....
Are (were) you close? **1.** **2.** **3.** **0.** (does not know) ←

Given name : .... **Sex :** F2 M1 **Age :** |__|__| **or year of birth:** |__|__|__|__|
Child of: ....
Frequency of contact: .... Lives with you
Does this child ever stay into your home without the parents? **1.** Yes **2.** No
How often or on what occasions? ....
....
Are (were) you close? **1.** **2.** **3.** **0.** (does not know) ←

Given name : .... **Sex :** F2 M1 **Age :** |__|__| **or year of birth:** |__|__|__|__|
Child of: ....
Frequency of contact: .... Lives with you
Does this child ever stay into your home without the parents? **1.** Yes **2.** No
How often or on what occasions? ....
....
Are (were) you close? **1.** **2.** **3.** **0.** (does not know) ←

Given name : .... **Sex :** F2 M1 **Age :** |__|__| **or year of birth:** |__|__|__|__|
Child of: ....
Frequency of contact: .... Lives with you
Does this child ever stay into your home without the parents? **1.** Yes **2.** No
How often or on what occasions? ....
....
Are (were) you close? **1.** **2.** **3.** **0.** (does not know) ←

Given name : .... **Sex :** F2 M1 **Age :** |__|__| **or year of birth:** |__|__|__|__|
Child of: ....
Frequency of contact: .... Lives with you
Does this child ever stay into your home without the parents? **1.** Yes **2.** No
How often or on what occasions? ....
....
Are (were) you close? **1.** **2.** **3.** **0.** (does not know) ←

Beside the family members whom we just talked about, are there other persons, friends or family, who have played an important role for you, favorably or not.

Given name	Sex F M	Age difference	Your relation with this person?	Why was this person important to you In what way positively or not?	
1. When you were a child (at school, in the neighbourhood...)					
....	2 1	+ = -	....	....	☐
....	2 1	+ = -	....	....	☐
....	2 1	+ = -	....	....	☐
....	2 1	+ = -	....	....	☐
....	2 1	+ = -	....	....	☐
....	2 1	+ = -	....	....	☐
2. When you were a teenager (at school, in the neighbourhood...)					
....	2 1	+ = -	....	....	☐
....	2 1	+ = -	....	....	☐
....	2 1	+ = -	....	....	☐
....	2 1	+ = -	....	....	☐
....	2 1	+ = -	....	....	☐
....	2 1	+ = -	....	....	☐
....	2 1	+ = -	....	....	☐

Given name	Sex F M	Age difference	Your relation with this person?	Why was this person important to you? In what way? Positively or not?	
3. When you were a young adult (during your studies, at work...)					
....	2 1	+ = -	....	....	☐
....	2 1	+ = -	....	....	☐
....	2 1	+ = -	....	....	☐
....	2 1	+ = -	....	....	☐
....	2 1	+ = -	....	....	☐
....	2 1	+ = -	....	....	☐
....	2 1	+ = -	....	....	☐
....	2 1	+ = -	....	....	☐
....	2 1	+ = -	....	....	☐
4. As an adult (when you started a family, at work...)					
....	2 1	+ = -	....	....	☐
....	2 1	+ = -	....	....	☐
....	2 1	+ = -	....	....	☐
....	2 1	+ = -	....	....	☐
....	2 1	+ = -	....	....	☐
....	2 1	+ = -	....	....	☐
....	2 1	+ = -	....	....	☐
....	2 1	+ = -	....	....	☐
....	2 1	+ = -	....	....	☐
....	2 1	+ = -	....	....	☐
....	2 1	+ = -	....	....	☐
....	2 1	+ = -	....	....	☐
5. Now					
....	2 1	+ = -	....	....	☐
....	2 1	+ = -	....	....	☐
....	2 1	+ = -	....	....	☐
....	2 1	+ = -	....	....	☐
....	2 1	+ = -	....	....	☐
....	2 1	+ = -	....	....	☐
....	2 1	+ = -	....	....	☐
....	2 1	+ = -	....	....	☐
....	2 1	+ = -	....	....	☐
....	2 1	+ = -	....	....	☐
....	2 1	+ = -	....	....	☐

Among these people, who are those whom you consider as close? (*tick the box in the column*)

Now let us try to map out your own residential and occupational history

THE FAMILY CODES
MUST BE ENTERED IN THE
"FAMILY" COLUMN OF THE GRID

Counting all sources:

salaries, wages end/or sellf-employment income

revenue from public sources (e.g;, child tax benefits, employement insurance benefits, Canada or Québec pension plan benefits, old age security benefits)

revenue from interest, dividents or other investments

revenue from private pension plan

alimony payments

other revenue

What is your best estimate of the total revenue (before deductions) of all members of your household, from all sources, over the last 12 months?

R1 Unprompted response: .... per year

R2 *(if not, offer the following choises)*

1. less than $5,000

2. between $5,000 and $10,000

3. between $10,000 and $15,000

4. between $15,000 and $20,000

5. between $20,000 and $25,000

6. between $25,000 and $30,000

7. between $30,000 and $40,000

8. between $40,000 and $50,000

9. between $50,000 and $60,000

10. between $60,000 and $75,000

11. over $75,000

00. Does not know

F1 **Do you intend to move house?**

1. Yes **2.** Maybe **3.** No

F2 **Why?** ....

....

....

....

....

F3 **Where (municipality, province, region, be specific)?**

....

Would you agree to be contacted again by a researcher of our team for an open interview on a similar subject?

1. Yes **2.** No

Tkank you for your cooperation

Interview end time |__|__|__|__|

References

Attias-Donfut, C. (Ed.). (1995). *Les solidarités entre générations: vieillesse, familles, État*. Paris: Nathan, coll. "Essais et recherche", série Sciences sociales.

Attias-Donfut, C., Lapierre, N., & Segalen, M. (2002). *Le nouvel esprit de famille. Enquête trigénérationnelle*. Paris: Éditions Odile Jacob.

Axinn, W. G., Barber, J. S., & Ghimire, D. J. (1997). The neighbourhood history calendar: A data collection method designed for multilevel modelling. *Sociological Methodology, 27*, 355–392.

Bastide, H., & Girard, A. (1974). Mobilité résidentielle de la population et motivations des personnes: une enquête auprès du public. II, Les motifs de la mobilité. *Population, 29*(4–5), 743–769.

Bastide, H., & Girard, A. (1975). Attitudes et opinions des Français à l'égard de la fécondité et de la famille. *Population, 30*(4–5), 693–749.

Bengtson, V.-L., & Roberts, R. E.-L. (1991). Intergenerational solidarity in aging families: An example of formal theory construction. *Journal of Marriage and the Family, 53*(4), 856–870.

Berger, M. (2004). *Les péri-urbains de Paris. De la ville dense à la métropole*. Paris: CNRS Éditions.

Bertillon, J. (1894). *Essai de statistique comparée du surpeuplement des habitations à Paris et dans les grandes capitales européennes*. Paris: Imprimerie Chaix.

Bonvalet, C. (1987). Les Parisiens dans leur maturité: origine, parcours, intégration. *Population, 42*(2), 225–247.

Bonvalet, C. (Ed.). (1994). *Logement, mobilité et populations urbaines*. Paris: CNRS Éditions, PirVilles.

Bonvalet, C. (2003). The local family circle. *Population, English Edition, 58*(1), 9–42.

Bonvalet, C., & Gotman, A. (Eds.). (1993). *Le logement, une affaire de famille: L'approche intergénérationnelle des statuts résidentiels* (168 p.). Paris: L'Harmattan.

Bonvalet, C., & Lelièvre, E. (1989). La mobilité résidentielle en France et à Paris depuis 1945. 1) Bilan résidentiel d'une génération. *Population, 44*(3), 531–560.

Bonvalet, C., & Lelièvre, E. (1991a). Nuptialité et mobilité. In T. Hibert & L. Roussel (Eds.), *La Nuptialité: évolution récente en France et dans les pays développés* (pp. 237–253). Paris: INED.

Bonvalet, C., & Lelièvre, E. (1991b). Mobilité en France et à Paris depuis 1945. Le filtre parisien. *Population, 46*(5), 1161–1184.

Bonvalet, C., & Lelièvre, E., (1995a, 27 August–3 September). *La notion d'entourage, un outil pour l'analyse de l'évolution des réseaux individuels*, Paper presented at 18th International Congress of Historical Sciences, Montreal, INED, Dossiers et recherches, 52, Paris.

Bonvalet, C., & Lelièvre, E. (1995b). Du concept de ménage à celui d'entourage: une redéfinition de l'espace familial. *Sociologie et Societes, 27*(2), 177–190.

Bonvalet, C., & Lelièvre, E. (Eds.). (2012). De la famille à l'entourage, Collection Les Grandes Enquêtes, Ed. de l'Ined/PUF, Paris, 472 p.

Bonvalet, C., Maison, D., Le Bras, H., & Charles, L. (1993). Proches et parents. *Population, 48*(1), 83–110.

Bonvalet, C., Gotman, A., & Grafmeyer, Y. (Eds.). (2007). *Family kinship and place in France* (244 p.). London: Southern Universities Press.

Bott, E. (1957). *Family and social network*. London: Tavistock.

Chevalier, L. (1950). *La formation de la population parisienne au 19ème siècle*. Paris: INED/PUF.

Chombart de Lauwe, P. H. (1956). *La vie quotidienne des familles ouvrières. Recherches sur les comportements sociaux de consommation*. Paris: CNRS.

Cicchelli-Pugeault, C., & Cicchelli, V. (1998). *Les théories sociologiques de la famille* (p. 236). Paris: La Découverte, coll. "Repères".

Clerc, P. (1967). *Grands ensembles, banlieues nouvelles. Enquête démographique et psychosociologique*. Paris: INED/PUF, Cahier Travaux et documents, 49.

Coenen-Huther, J., Kellerhals, J., & Von Allmen, M. (1994). *Les réseaux de solidarité dans la famille*. Lausanne: Éditions Réalités sociales.
Courgeau, D. (1984). Relations entre cycle de vie et migrations. *Population, 39*(3), 483–514.
Courgeau, D. (1985). Interaction between spatial mobility, family and career life-cycle: A French survey. *European Sociological Review, 1*(2), 139–162.
Courgeau, D. (1987). Constitution de la famille et urbanisation. *Population, 42*(1), 57–82.
Courgeau, D., & Lelièvre, E. (1986). Nuptialité et agriculture. *Population, 41*(2), 303–326.
Crenner, E. (1998). *La parenté: un réseau de sociabilité actif mais concentré*. Insee Première, 600.
Crenner, E. (1999). *Famille, je vous aide*. Insee Première, 631.
Cribier, F., & Kych, A. (1992). La migration de retraite des Parisiens: une analyse de la propension au départ. *Population, 47*(3), 677–718.
Cribier, F., Duffau, M. L., & Kych, A. (1990). Mobilité résidentielle et stratégie dans les quinze ans qui suivent la retraite: suivi d'une génération, *Stratégies résidentielles*. Paris: INED, coll. "Congrès et colloques", 2, pp. 283–296.
Dandurand, R.-B., & Ouellette, F.-R. (1992). *Entre autonomie et solidarités. Parenté et soutien dans la vie des jeunes familles montréalaises*. Québéc: INRS Culture et société.
Déchaux, J.-H. (2003). La parenté dans les sociétés occidentales modernes: un éclairage structural. *Recherches et Prévisions, 72*, 53–63.
de Tocqueville, A. (1835). *De la démocratie en Amérique*. Paris: Flammarion.
Garigue, P. (1956). French Canadian kinship and urban life. *American Anthropologist, 58*, 1090–1101.
Girard, A. (1974). *Le choix du conjoint*. Paris: INED, coll. "Travaux et Documents", Cahier 70.
Girard, A., & Bastide, H. (1952). Enquête sur le logement des jeunes ménages dans le département de la Seine. *Population, 7*(4), 617–636.
Girard, A., & Zucker, E. (1968). La conjoncture démographique: régulation des naissances, famille et natalité: une enquête auprès du public. *Population, 23*(2), 225–264.
Gokalp, C. (1978). Le réseau familial. *Population, 33*(6), 1077–1094.
Grab (Groupe de réflexion sur l'approche biographique), 2009 (1st ed. 1999), *Biographies d'enquêtes, bilan de 14 collectes biographiques*. Paris: INED, coll. "Méthodes et Savoirs", 3, 340p. grab.site.ined.fr/fr/editions_en_ligne/biographies_enquetes/
Hammer, R., Burton-Jeangros, C., & Kellerhalls, J. (2001). Le lien de parenté dans les jeunes générations suisses: lignées, structures et fonctions. *Population, 56*(4), 515–538.
Henry, L. (1949). Structure de la population et besoins de logements. *Population, 4*(3), 433–446.
Henry, L. (1950). Perspectives relatives aux besoins de logements. *Population, 5*(3), 493–512.
Héran, F. (1982). Cycle de vie et cycle des relations de parenté. In *Les Âges de la vie*, actes du VIIe colloque national de démographie. Paris: INED, Vol. I, coll. "Travaux et documents", cahier 96.
Heran, F. (1987). *"Les relations de voisinage", Données Sociales*. Paris: INSEE.
Kempeneers, M., Lelievre, E., & Bonvalet, C. (2007). Benefits of a longitudinal approach in family solidarity surveys: Reflections on the temporal nature of exchanges. *Canadian Studies in Population, 34*(1), 69–83.
Lelièvre, E. (1990). Point des connaissances quantitatives en matière de mobilité résidentielle. In *Stratégies résidentielles*. Paris: INED, Congrès et Colloques, 2, pp. 73–84.
Lelièvre, E., & Bonvalet, C. (1994). A compared cohort history of residential mobility, social change and home-ownership in Paris and the rest of France. *Urban Studies, 31*(10), 1647–1666.
Lelièvre, E., & Vivier, G. (2001). Évaluation d'une collecte à la croisée du quantitatif et du qualitatif, l'enquête Biographies et entourage. *Population, 56*(6), 1043–1073.
Lelievre, E., Bonvalet, C., & Bry, X. (1997). Event history analysis of groups. The findings of an on-going research project. *Population, An English Selection*, special issue: *New methodological approaches in the social sciences, 110*(1), 11–37.
Litwak, E. (1985). *Helping the elderly. The complementary roles of informal networks and formal systems*. New York: The Guildford Press.

Michel, A. (1955). La population des hôtels meublés à Paris: composition et conditions d'existence. *Population, 10*(4), 627–644.
Michel, A. (1970a). *La sociologie de la famille*. Paris: Mouton.
Michel, A. (1970b). La famille urbaine et la parenté. In R. König & R. Hill (Eds.), *Family in east and west*. Paris: Mouton.
Ortalda, L. (2001). *Le système d'entraide au sein de la parenté: entre logiques sociales et pratiques familiales*. PhD thesis, université Paris-X Nanterre.
Parsons, T. (1955). The kinship system of the contemporary United State. In F. Bourricaud (Ed.), *Éléments pour une sociologie de l'action*. Paris: Plon.
Pilon, M., & Vignikin, K. (2007). *Ménages et familles en Afrique subsaharienne*. Paris: Éditions des Archives contemporaines. coll. "Savoirs francophones".
Pitrou, A. (1972). *La famille dans la vie de tous les jours?* Toulouse: Privat.
Pitrou, A. (1978). *Vivre sans famille? Les solidarités familiales dans le monde d'aujourd'hui*. Toulouse: Privat.
Poulain, M., Riandey, B., & Firdion, J. M. (1991). Enquête biographique et registre belge de population: confrontation des données. *Population, 46*(1), 65–88.
Pourcher, G. (1963). Le peuplement de Paris. Origine régionale, composition sociale, attitudes et motivations. Présentation d'une enquête de l'Ined et de la préfecture de la Seine. *Population, 18*(3), 545–564.
Pourcher, G. (1964). Le peuplement de Paris: origine régionale, composition sociale, attitudes et motivations, Paris, Ined, coll. "Travaux et documents", 43.
Pourcher, G. (1966). Un essai d'analyse par cohorte de la mobilité géographique et professionnelle. *Population, 21*(2), 356–378.
Pourcher, G., Bastide, H., & Girard, A. (1964). Mobilité géographique et concentration urbaine en France: une enquête en province. *Population, 19*(2), 227–266.
Rémy, J. (1967). Persistance de la famille étendue dans un milieu industriel et urbain. *Revue française de sociologie, 8*(4), 493–505.
Roussel, L., with Odile Bourguignon. (1976). *La famille après le mariage des enfants: étude des relations entre générations*. Paris: INED, coll "Travaux et documents", 78.
Sauvy, A. (1946). Logement et population. *Population, 1*(3), 441–452.
Segalen, M. (1981). *Sociologie de la famille*. Paris, Armand Colin 6e édition révisée et augmentée. Paris: Armand Colin, 2006.
Segalen, M. (2006)/ (1e éd. 1981). Sociologie de la famille, Paris, Armand Colin, Paris.
Sussman, M.-B. (1959). The isolated nuclear family: Fact or fiction? *Social Problems, 6*, 333–339.
Sussman, M. B., & Burchinal, L. (1962). Kin family network: heared structure in current conceptualizations of family functioning". *Marriage and Family Living, 24*(3), 231–240.
Tabard, N. (1993a). *Représentation socioéconomique du territoire: typologie des quartiers et communes selon la profession et l'activité économique de leurs habitants. France métropolitaine, recensement de 1990* (Direction des statistiques démographiques et sociales). Paris: INSEE, Documents de travail F/9304.
Tabard, N. (1993b). Des quartiers pauvres aux banlieues crisées: une représentation sociale du territoire. *Economie et statistique, 270*, 5–22.
Willmott, P. (2007). Preface to English edition. In C. Bonvalet, A. Gotman, & Y. Grafmeyer (Eds.), *Family, kinship and place in France*. London: Southern Universities Press.
Young, M., & Willmott, P. (1957). *Family and kinship in east London*. London: Routledge and Kegan Paul.
Zarca, B. (1993a). L'héritage de l'indépendance professionnelle selon les lignées, le sexe et le rang dans la fratrie. *Population, 48*(2), 275–306.
Zarca, B. (1993b). L'Héritage de l'indépendance professionnelle : un ou plusieurs élus au sein de la fratrie? *Population, 48*(4), 1015–1042.

Chapter 3
A Conceptual Shift from "Household" to "Entourage": Redefining the Scope of the Family

Catherine Bonvalet and Éva Lelièvre

The changes in society over the past several decades have prompted a number of researchers to question the analytical tools and categories used to describe the "new social morphology". In the area of family studies, demographers have a range of traditional tools and concepts at their disposal. However, while these are necessary for analysing changing family structures, they present certain limitations when it comes to describing family reality.

In most economic and socio-demographic studies, "the household" is the main concept used by statisticians, demographers and economists to link the family to other areas, such as consumption, housing and infrastructure. On the face of it, there is nothing problematic about using the term "household"; as Alain Desrosières puts it, we "don't question something unquestionable" (1993). But attempts to develop a dynamic approach to new socio-demographic configurations reveal the ambiguity and limitations of the terms "family" and "household", creating tension between the available data, the operationality of the analytical categories and their conceptual – and even semantic – imprecision. Alain Desrosières describes this tension aptly: "the space of statistical information is particularly important if we want to explore what makes a public space both possible and impossible.[1] The tension between the fact that statistical data purport to be a reference in public debate while at the same time being constantly open to question, and hence themselves a potential subject of the debate, is a major difficulty when it comes to conceptualizing the conditions in which such a space might be possible".

[1] A. Desrosières (1993) defines "the public space as a space within which issues facing a community can be made the subject of public debate, partly in conjunction with the existence of statistical data that is accessible to all".

This article first appeared in the journal *Sociologie et sociétés*, 1995, 27(2), pp. 177–190.

C. Bonvalet (✉) • É. Lelièvre (✉)
Institut national d'études démographiques (INED), Paris, France
e-mail: bonvalet@ined.fr; eva@ined.fr

C. Bonvalet, É. Lelièvre (eds.), *Family Beyond Household and Kin*,
INED Population Studies 6, DOI 10.1007/978-3-319-24684-0_3

In the socio-demographic literature, two concepts are used to describe family configurations: "the household" and "the family". They became interchangeable in the post-war period, when the nuclear family, which conforms exactly to the statistical unit of the household, emerged as the universal family model. But the two concepts are starting to come apart at the seams. For a start, neither adequately describes the reality of families, i.e. the mobility and social reproduction strategies implemented within the kin network. Furthermore, for census purposes, in France (and many other countries), the definition of a "family" is based on co-residence, which has sustained the confusion between "the family" and "the household".[2]

As Jean-Louis Flandrin reminds us, in the sixteenth, seventeenth and eighteenth centuries, "the concept of family could refer either to co-residence or to kinship, two ideas that are conflated in the definition most commonly used today. In past centuries, the word 'family' was used much more frequently to refer to a group of relatives who did not live together, but was also commonly used for a set of people who lived together but were not necessarily related by blood or marriage" (Flandrin 1976). It was not until the nineteenth century that living together and being closely related merged into a single concept of "family".

This confusion between family and household that causes conceptual vagueness can be attributed largely to the available data. According to the most common statistical definition, a family is defined as persons related by filiation or marriage who co-reside. Divorced parents who share custody of their children, with the children alternating between each parent's home, are not considered a family because they represent more than one household.

This research has two objectives: to reconnect members of the household with the family group in order to understand its role in the social strategies of individuals, and to reintroduce the time element in order to understand the dynamics of these processes.

The event-history approach adopted here seeks to go beyond the traditional view of households and families with a view to examining changes in the family group and its individual members over a lifetime. Indeed, it was this approach that led researchers to reformulate the basis of demographic analysis in terms of complex stochastic processes (Courgeau and Lelièvre 1989). Each individual's life course is repositioned in the broadest possible context and the analysis of each demographic event can thus take into account adjacent or concurrent processes that the individual might be experiencing at the same point in time. Examining the dynamics of family groups involves observing the change between time t and time $t+1$, as well as analysing variations in family size and composition over time. Our approach thus necessarily involves the univocal identification of a changing entity of variable size

[2] It cannot be denied that statistical institutions play a role in the construct of the "family". Pierre Bourdieu (1993) writes: "the dominant, legitimate definition of a normal family (which may be explicit, as it is in law, or implicit, in for example the family questionnaires produced by state statistical agencies) is based on a constellation of words – *house*, *home*, *household*, which, while seeming to describe social reality, in fact construct it. On this definition, a family is a set of related individuals linked either by alliance (marriage) or filiation, or, less commonly, by adoption, and living under the same roof (co-residence)".

and composition. While the history of families is concerned with conjugal and filial ties that change as individuals progress through life, the history of households occurs at the intersection of the history of individuals and the history of places. By identifying its significant agents, this research will seek to identify the entourage that influences and is influenced by the individual. The hypothesis here is that an individual's life course is shaped – to a varying extent depending on the person and the period – by the influences of other individuals upon him or her and, conversely, by the influence he/she has on those other individuals.

This is an attempt at a *construct* that dissociates the dynamics of the entourage from the individuals themselves, with the aim of measuring the following:

1. The influence of the individual on the group;
2. The influence of the group on the individual.

These two elements will be measured by an individual's *position* within the circle of their close relatives and by the *type(s) of co-residence* experienced by the individual, both past and present.

In a demographic study of this kind, the individual's influence on the group is manifested, for example, in his/her propensity to increase the size of the group (by becoming a parent, for example) or in his/her mobility if this causes other people to move and results in a spatial reorganization of the network of close relatives. In turn, an individual's mode of co-residence (living with parents, friends, or children) influences his/her mobility, fertility, etc. The system of influences is thus built upon the successive households to which an individual has belonged (assuming the individual has co-resided with others), and upon key individuals external to these households, on the basis of ties centred on marriage or filiation. This makes up an individual's "entourage". To take the methodological exploration further, we need to review both the concepts and the data at our disposal. This chapter therefore begins with a critical review of the concepts of "family" and "household" with the aim of better defining the concept of "entourage". It goes on to analyse the data on family relationships available at a given point in time, as well as data on the changes that occur in the domestic group over the course of its existence. These findings will then be used to justify our concept of "the entourage", and the terms of its analysis.

3.1 Which Should Take Priority: Families or Households?

3.1.1 Limitations of the Concepts of "Household" and "Family"

We shall begin by examining the definitions of a household. Defined in France as a group of individuals living under the same roof, a household is a statistical entity measured at a particular moment in time and based on a residence criterion. In other words, it is a cross-sectional unit, the characteristics of which are observed at a single, specific moment in time. The household is the most complex primary unit of analysis linking individuals (Kuijsten and Vossen 1988) and can describe any number of scenarios, ranging from a single person living alone to a group of unrelated people living under the same roof, via a co-resident family.

In terms of data collection, the concept of household, in cross-sectional studies at least, appears to be quite functional. The household is an easily identifiable group at a given point in time and represents the essential unit for major national surveys such as censuses and labour surveys and household surveys in general. This means that information is available on the structure of households at least, making it possible to compare situations at different dates. However, a household is a complex statistical unit with socioeconomic characteristics, which may be defined in different countries on the basis of one or more of the following:

1. location
2. household members' relationships
3. shared lifestyle, especially shared daily meals or shared living room
4. joint income
5. joint consumption

In industrialized countries, the household may refer to two concepts: the household as an economic unit and the household as a housing unit. Under the first definition, a single dwelling may contain two economic units (for instance, a family with a lodger occupying one room of their house/apartment without a shared lifestyle). If the household is defined as a housing unit, however, a single dwelling can contain only one household.[3]

Clearly, the concept of household is highly complex. The difficulties described above are compounded by the existence, it seems to us, of three distinct objectives in the household-as-housing-unit approach:

1. To provide a description of housing stock[4] by distinguishing between primary residences, secondary residences and vacant dwellings in successive censuses in order to track changes in housing conditions or occupancy status (e.g. the rate of home-ownership among different social classes);
2. To identify the relevant decision-making entity in a group of individuals with a view to studying how choices are made with respect to housing, acquisition of durable goods and consumption. In economics, a household is thus defined as a unit of consumption, a definition that considers not only the size of the household but also the age of its members;
3. To provide a description of family systems with a view to capturing the family "concealed" in the statistics. To this end, the different types of family that a

[3] "In France the definition of a household fits that of a dwelling just like a snail fits its shell." (Le Bras 1979)

[4] "A 'household' will soon be interchangeable with a dwelling which, under the influence of hygienists and property speculators, is becoming a statistical unit. We count the number of kitchens, rooms, conveniences and we fit the 'household' into it without any further detail than a headcount of its members.", Le Bras, *op. cit.*

household may include are identified by defining the primary family and, in some cases, the secondary family – in the latter case, a biological nucleus may be reconstructed by analysing the relationship between the various household members and the household reference person.

The second and third objectives seem hard to attain when the entity of the household is used, i.e. when the definition of a household is restricted to co-residence. This approach to the question of families is not new. The following two typologies, which illustrate the common conceptual conflation of household and family, show that studying social and family morphology using the household as a unit of analysis is also problematic for studying societies of the past.

Le Play (1871) was a forerunner in the development of family typologies. He made a meticulous examination of family life and converted daily routines into figures by drawing up family budgets. Based on these "monographs", Le Play identified several categories of family (Le Play 1901). His three main family types include two extreme types – the patriarchal family and the unstable family – and one intermediate type – the stem family:

1. A patriarchal family is one in which all the sons, married or unmarried, live in the paternal home and property remains undivided between the members of the family. In Le Play's view, a patriarchal family "both in its work regimen and social relations, values attachment to the past over concern with the future, and obedience over initiative";
2. An unstable family is one where the children leave their parents' home once they become financially independent and form unstable families of their own. "The proliferation of unstable families on bare cleared land consigns a dispossessed populace to a perpetual state of suffering. It gives rise to these sinister metropolises never before seen in history";
3. In a stem family (*famille souche*), only one of the children stays with the parents, living with them as well as with their own children. "In the paternal home, the stem family retains all the habits of working life, the means to prosper, and the treasury of valuable lessons handed down from forebears. The stem family becomes a permanent haven, to which any member of the family can turn in times of hardship. By virtue of these traditions, the stem family provides individuals with a degree of security not found in unstable families and a degree of independence incompatible with patriarchal ones".

We shall not revisit the debates sparked by Le Play's theories. We shall simply note Peter Laslett's criticism of the evolutionist views of theorists from Le Play to Parsons, which attribute the disappearance of complex structures to industrial progress and individualism (Parsons and Bales, 1955). Laslett refutes the universality of the nuclear family today and the belief that extended families were the past norm, maintaining that the phenomenon of the nuclear family is not a consequence of industrialization and urbanisation but has in fact always existed (Flandrin 1976).

Laslett defines a simple-family household as a nuclear family, an elementary family or a biological family, whose nucleus is a married couple living together. An enlarged family consists of this conjugal family unit plus other close kin. Lastly, an extended family is the full set of related individuals who maintain close relations but do not live together. Laslett (1972, p. 31) uses the expression households and proposes the following typology:

1. "Solitaries" and "no family" domestic groups consisting of a single person (such as widows) or co-resident siblings, relatives of other kinds or unrelated co-residents;
2. "Simple family" households corresponding to the contemporary family unit. These consist of either a couple and their children (nuclear family), or a widowed or separated parent and his/her children;
3. "Extended family" households consisting of members of a simple domestic group together with ascendants, descendants and collateral relatives;
4. "Multiple family" household, where several related families co-reside. This category can be further divided, according to the status of the household head. If authority is held by the senior couple, with married children deferring to a paternal authority figure, the model corresponds to Le Play's stem family. A family consisting of siblings and their spouses all belonging to the same generation is described as a *frérèche*.

The aim of this review of the terminology is not to challenge the household as a concept per se but, on the contrary, to clarify its usage in order to avoid semantic drift. The question to be asked when the term "household" is used to study families is what type of family it refers to.

Indeed, the term "family" does not refer solely to parent-child relationships. It refers more broadly to individuals related by blood and marriage no matter how distant they may be, e.g. second cousins. Without wanting to question the statistical approach, limited by the availability of data, the point can nevertheless be made that in defining families by household, we deny the very thing that constitutes family, i.e. family ties. In France, a widow and her grandson are not considered a family, whereas a cohabiting couple is, regardless of how long the partners have been together (perhaps only 2 months at the time a census was taken). The ties between collateral relatives are not recognized: for example, two brothers living together would be considered as "a non-family household".

To sum up, the real problem is the emphasis on residence in the definition of a family – because the term "family", which may mean a number of things, is confusing – and consequently in the way that families are analysed. In statistical studies, the description of family structures drawn from census data is often used as the basis for analysing families (Villac 1991; Durr 1991). This approach involves a not insignificant risk of equating families with households (Audirac 1985), in other words reducing families to the statistical unit found in surveys and censuses. From this point of view, a family is seen as a sub-unit of a household (Lefranc 1995), when in fact the terms could be reversed and a household could be thought of as being a sub-unit of a family.

3.1.2 A New Concept: The Entourage

The foregoing discussion of various typologies and how they have been used to study family forms has highlighted the limitations of the available concepts for analysing these structures. The two concepts, both delimited by the framework of co-residence, ignore the influence of an individual's network. We therefore argue that family ties beyond the household be taken into account and added to the concept of "the household" to eliminate the problematic ambiguity and semantic drift that we have identified with respect to the terms "family" and "household". This new conceptual infrastructure, which we are naming "entourage" and which may at first glance seem less workable than the other two more commonly used terms, actually clarifies analysis by distinguishing clearly between the sphere of influence of people who live under the same roof and that of people who are related by marriage or blood, which may extend beyond the household. One of the advantages of the term "entourage" is that it is not restricted to either co-residents or to relatives. The theoretical construct that we are proposing seeks not only to describe this system of influence at a specific point in time but also allows us to follow changes in this structure over time.

The complexity of the object of analysis, especially in its longitudinal dimension, means that any descriptive portrayal of the changes to an individual's entourage will require – at least at the outset – several simplifying hypotheses to make it operational. To this end, we propose the following definitions:

- *The position* of the individual may be described schematically in terms of whether he/she is related (blood relationship) or whether he/she is in a couple or not (whether there is a revocable conjugal bond or not), under the criteria identified by Henry (1972) and adopted by Ryder (1985);
- *The types of co-residence* experienced by an individual are very diverse in nature and will be culturally marked. We might limit ourselves to identifying basic types, such as whether one lives with one's parents, one's children, in a conjugal relationship or alone. To this should be added more complex situations, such as living with peers (including collateral relatives) and living simultaneously with children and parents or peers, or with non-relatives, etc.;
- *The "minimum" entourage* thus consists of all of the household members plus any non-cohabiting children of the individual and his/her cohabiting partner. This model retains two fundamental aspects of family: filiation (of direct descent) and conjugal relationships (initially, only conjugal relationships between cohabiting partners are used in this definition). The definition also includes the individual's domestic group (people living with him/her).

The portrayal soon becomes more complicated if the following non-cohabitants are included in the entourage: parents (the other form of direct descent), financial and emotional dependents, and significant others, with these last two categories falling outside the traditional scope of demography.

Roles combine in complex ways. Parent-child relationships endure regardless of changes in conjugal relationships (successive unions) or changes in place of residence. With this in mind, we will endeavour to gather information about the parent of a respondent's children who is no longer cohabiting, even when the two partners have separated. On the other hand, if we proceed on the basis of the equality of individuals in conjugal relationships in the sense that, once a childless union has ended, the separated partners no longer have any obligations with respect to each other, we would not follow an individual's ex-partner. Under this convention, it is only the responsibilities conferred by filiation that would persist as significant ties. In a longitudinal study of an individual's entourage, it would be appropriate to keep a record of all relatives of direct descent because we assume they have an influence on the individual's behaviour and, conversely, that the individual has a major determining impact on those persons' lives, whether they live together or not. Making this assumption requires a degree of "memory loss" with regard to past unions that did not produce children and amounts to "just keeping the children".[5] This reflects the asymmetry between conjugal and filial relationships.

Not only would this new concept get around the problem of semantic drift that we have identified in the use of the terms "family" and "household", but it would also serve as a new methodological infrastructure offering an alternative reading to the conventional view of the two types of "family crisis", by postulating that these so-called crises are primarily changes in modes of co-residence:

- the transition from the complex family to the nuclear family, deplored by Le Play and the moralists of the nineteenth century, a crusade taken up again by T. Parsons in the US in 1955[6];
- the subsequent decline in the proportion of nuclear families with the rise in the number of solitaries and of non-marital unions, and the increase in divorces and separations.[7]

In either of these two cases, one may challenge the assertion that the family (in the sense of the "extended family" as defined by Peter Laslett) has undergone a profound crisis,[8] even if periods of mass migration have, in the immediate term, loosened the ties between related individuals.

---

[5] This implies, in terms of longitudinal data collection, that in case of a young woman's history, we would include the first instance of her living with a partner and the characteristics of that partner for the duration of their cohabitation. If they were to separate without having had any children, we would cease to gather information on the young man's subsequent life. If a short time later the young woman was to form a couple with a man who had children from a previous union, we would include details about those children and thus, incidentally, details about the former partner of the young woman's new partner.

[6] The authors (Parsons and Bales) describe the structural isolation of the modern family and the breakdown in inter-generational ties, which leads to the abandonment of moral and family values and the failure to pass on family assets.

[7] Monique Buisson and Jean-Claude Mermet (1988) have shown that separation does not automatically destroy the couple's role as parents: "Pratiques sociales de l'habitat et dynamiques de la divortialité", in *Transformations de la famille et habitat* (C. Bonvalet, P. Merlin, eds.), Paris, INED, DREIF, IDEF, *Travaux et Documents*, 120, 1988.

[8] In response to criticisms of his theory drawing parallels between the nuclear family and aspects of urban industrial society, T. Parsons made the clarification that the concept of the nuclear family

These different interpretations of the evolution of family structures make it clear that, to avoid confusion, we need to exercise caution when using the terms "household" and "family". As we have seen with Le Play, the ambiguity frequently seen in articles and books often has ideological and moral connotations. These connotations may be unconscious, but language is not neutral.[9]

On the basis of broad family types, a hierarchy of family ties can be established – supposedly strong in complex households and weak in nuclear or single-family households. It is only through an understanding of the entourage that we can determine the strength, the role and the persistence over time of relationships between both cohabitants and non-cohabitants.

At this point in our analysis, it is clear that the household is not really the appropriate unit for observing families. With divorces, separations and various complex situations of semi co-residence, the statistical concept of the household is increasingly at odds with the realities of family and social life that it is supposed to describe. Social reality falls somewhere in between the domestic group of co-residents and the complete extended family. It is the full set of households associated with a given family network and their members that form the resource available to individuals, with which they interact in order to have and raise children, to navigate the housing and labour markets, to move around the country, and so on.

3.2 The Available Data

Surveys that have gathered data on the nature of networks of friends and family have either been a snapshot of the network at a given point in time[10] or an attempt at mapping specific types of relationship over a longer period (for example, surveys on the history of sexual partners).

---

was isolated in structural terms (quoted in Segalen 1993). Numerous studies, particularly from the United States and the United Kingdom, have subsequently shown that nuclear families were not isolated (Caplow et al. 1982; Young and Willmott 1957).

[9] The expression "single-parent family" is an interesting example. As Nadine Le Faucheur writes in an article in the journal *Dialogues* (No. 101, 1988), "this term seems to have the advantage of giving households headed by women the status of 'real families'. The negative connotation associated with these households until now has sometimes been reversed – not only are households headed by single women declared to be as normal as any other, they may sometimes even be presented as more 'modern' because they are more pioneering in terms of gender roles." In this case, the use of the word "family" is misleading and it would be more accurate to refer to "single-parent households" because the other parent is generally still around. Nadine Le Faucheur uses the term *famille bi-focale* – "two-home family" – in order not to disregard the absent parent in the way that the term "single-parent family" does (de Singly 1993), but even this solution does not seem to get around the problem of the confusion between "household" and "family" (Théry 1991). As Martine Segalen (1993) points out, in the case of stepfamilies, the concept of family is separated from that of co-residence. See also M. de Saboulin (1984, 1986).

[10] *Réseaux de Relations* survey, D. Courgeau (1972, 1975b); *Réseau familial* survey, C. Gokalp (1978); *Proches et parents* survey, C. Bonvalet, D. Maison, H. Le Bras and L. Charles et al. (1993).

3.2.1 A Cross-Sectional Study of Family Networks

The results of *Proches et parents* [Friends and family], a survey conducted by INED in 1990, suggest that it is possible to track an individual's entourage. If a count is made of all the relatives of two individuals living as a couple (including ascendants, descendants and collateral relatives), a high figure of around 40 is obtained, depending on the age of the individuals (Table 3.1). Variations in the extent and composition of the network of relatives also depend on the type of household the individual lives in. Even at the lower end of the scale, the figure for people who live alone can still be as high as 26. This shows that generally, without considering actual contact between the individual and his/her relatives, even people who live alone are not isolated in family terms.

By contrast, asking respondents to single out the people that they identify as their close family from the wider group of their relatives appears to narrow things down significantly. Even for couples with a network of around 40 people, the number of those identified as close family members is only around 5.5 on average, with young couples counting the highest number of relatives as close family (6.3), and older single men having the lowest number (2.8).

The limited number of persons identified as close family members within the extended family indicates that it would be quite practicable to reconstitute an individual's entourage. This would involve gathering a certain amount of retrospective information about the four or five people that the respondent identifies as close family. But before exploring the feasibility of this exercise further, let us review the longitudinal data that already exists.

In this area, even the most traditional surveys gather information on the respondent's partner and children, such as the dates of union formation and births. However, these data remain fragmentary. Surveys that have attempted to identify and follow

Table 3.1 Family network by age and household type in the *Proches et parents* survey (average number of people)

	Individual respondent's entire family network			
Respondent's status at the time of the survey	Living in a couple	Man living alone	Woman living alone	Single-parent family
Age				
Under 35	43.9	31.4	26.1	32.8
34–49	44.2	25.3	30.8	35.9
50–64	38.5	26.7	26.6	40.5
	Close family members			
Age				
Under 35	43.9	31.4	26.1	32.8
34–49	44.2	25.3	30.8	35.9
50–64	38.5	26.7	26.6	40.5
Over 64	4.9	2.8	3.5	5.2

Source: Bonvalet et al. 1993

the network of an individual respondent (the only realistic approach) have in fact gathered information about the composition of successive households the individual has been part of (as in the case of household panels such as in the Panel Study of Income Dynamics (PSID), Duncan and Morgan 1983).

While these examples do not map the entourage, they do provide scope for a more detailed examination of changes in social morphology and, more especially, their results confirm the need to go beyond the concepts of "household" and "family" that have been used to describe those changes. To illustrate what surveys of this kind can offer over and above the tables often compiled by juxtaposing statistics from successive censuses, we can look at the family histories of Parisians in 1986 through the prism of a survey called *Peuplement et dépeuplement de Paris* [Population and depopulation of Paris].

3.2.2 A Dynamic Study of Parisians' Domestic Histories

The data collected in the 1986 *Peuplement et dépeuplement* survey retraced the family and residential history of 1,987 residents of the Paris region aged 50–60. They were used to reconstruct the respondents' domestic histories from the time they became adults up to age 50.[11] These histories, which are an account of the different types of domestic group in which a person has lived, are by nature more complex than a person's marital history. Events that affect the composition of the domestic group involve not only the respondent but also any of the people with whom the respondent lives or has lived. Five types of household were recorded: single-person households; couples without children; couples with children; single-parent households; and complex households which were defined by the presence of ascendants or collateral relatives. Some 30 % of respondents began their adult lives living alone, 33 % in a couple and 35 % in a complex household[12] (Fig. 3.1).

Interestingly, the demographic history of these cohorts is often taken as the reference in demographic studies of fertility or divorce. These cohorts lived at a time when marriage was the near-universal norm, and the family model was that of the apparently "trouble-free" nuclear family, undisturbed by divorce or unmarried cohabitation. But although the demographic environment of the 1950s was still simple, economic conditions were not easy. These cohorts entered the housing market in the specific context of post-war France.

[11] 50 is the age at which we have a complete picture of the domestic histories of all of the respondents.

[12] One of the difficulties is to properly determine when "adult life" begins. The simplest solution would be to start at a fixed age for everybody, but this approach proves to be unsatisfactory due to the wide range of circumstances in which individuals leave home: from the apprentice who leaves his/her parents' home at age 14, to the young woman who marries at age 22, to the student who is still living at home at age 26. Another solution is to start with the respondent's first independent living arrangement, but this would exclude individuals who never move away from home. To resolve the issue, the survey designers considered that a respondent enters into adult life in one of three ways: by living independently, by marrying or, failing those two, after reaching age 25.

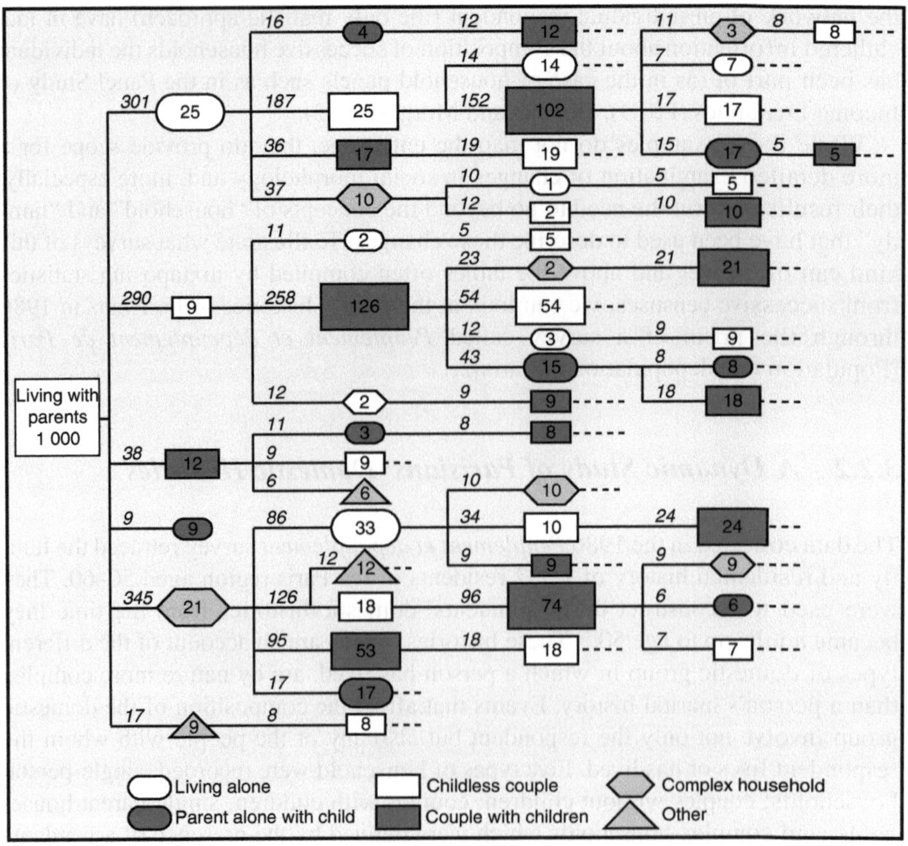

Fig. 3.1 Respondents' trajectories through family life from leaving their parents' home until age 50. *Interpretation*: The figures in *italics* represent flows: 301 people out of 1,000 who were living with their parents left to live on their own (i.e. 30 % of respondents initially moved out to live alone). The *boxed* figures represent the stock of people out of the initial 1,000 still living in that type of household at age 50, after having followed the previous pathway. For example, since leaving the parental home, 25 people were still living alone at age 50. The first pathway (at the *top* of the diagram) can be interpreted as follows: 301 people left home to live by themselves; out of those, 25 remained living alone, 16 subsequently lived alone with their children, 4 remained in that situation until age 50, while the 12 others formed a union with children and were still in that situation at age 50 (*Source*: *Peuplement et dépeuplement de Paris* survey, INED, 1986)

Considering these five types of household (six if you count 'other') and four stages in the domestic histories, a total of 1,296 routes are possible and no typical pattern appears. Importantly, the data do not overwhelmingly conform to the family history used as the reference in early demographic studies, namely: individuals leave their parents' home to get married, beginning their domestic life as a couple without children. This is followed by a period as a couple with children, then another period without children when the children in turn leave the parental home. Lastly, there is a stage of living alone after one member of the couple dies. Ending the period of observation at age 50 distorts the results, with the last two stages ("couple without children" and "person living alone") barely making an appearance. Some 13 % of respondents began living as a couple without children followed by a period living as a couple with children; and 11 % also experienced those two consecutive stages but after living alone initially. Adding a period of intergenerational co-residence at the beginning of both of the foregoing scenarios, all of these configurations together nevertheless account for 37 % of the respondents.

These few figures reveal the complexity of domestic histories. Beyond divorce or the death of a partner, both profoundly disruptive of the "traditional" family life cycle, other events – such as returning home to live with one's parents, or having a parent or sibling come to live in one's home, thus forming a complex household – are much more common than might be expected. It is certainly true that the vast majority of people – 8 out of 10 – have lived in a nuclear family at some point in their lives, but they got there in different ways (complex households, living alone, etc.). Equally, they left the "couple with children" stage in different ways. We observe, for example, that a number of people "skipped" the first two stages of the traditional family cycle, going directly from living with their parents to living in a nuclear family (either because the birth of their child occurred while the couple was still living with one or other of their families of origin, or because they married and had a child at around the same time). More than half of the men had lived alone for some period of their lives before age 50 compared with only 38 % of women. Around half of respondents had lived in a complex household (with ascendants or collateral relatives), which shows the significance of this form of co-residence that is now only marginally represented among the household structures recorded in the census. It is clear, however, that this phenomenon, which overwhelmingly occurs at the beginning of the respondents' adult lives, is related to the post-war historical context of housing shortage in the Paris region.

Despite relatively simple conjugal histories, these cohorts of Parisians lived in a wide variety of family structures. At each stage in their lives, the field of possibilities remained open. The fragility of unions and the proliferation of single-parent families and stepfamilies seen in younger cohorts has been reflected in increasingly complex domestic histories, and it will not be possible to effectively analyse these without additional information about key non-co-resident people in an individual's life.

A simple empirical description of the domestic histories of a cohort reveals the sheer complexity of individuals' life-courses. Moreover, the case we have presented does not take the time factor into account. Indeed, a large number of stages does not necessarily mean that each stage lasted only a short time; similarly, in a sequence with two stages, there is nothing in the description that indicates the amount of time spent in either stage.

The fact that a large number of individuals lived in a complex family at various times in their lives (Fig. 3.1) (returning to their family of origin, or providing a home for a parent or child) gives us an idea of the role of the extended family. But it is only a part of the picture because it is solely based on co-residence. Changes in emotional closeness and distance between family members are invisible to the analysis. The concept of "the entourage" would remove that limitation.

3.3 Conclusion

In the case of a longitudinal study, the combined notions of "household/family" discussed above do not seem to provide us with a workable concept. Indeed, what does following a complex group over time involve? It requires a definition that uniquely identifies the group over the course of time. The cross-sectional basis of the definition of a "household" – i.e. co-residence – does not work in a longitudinal analysis because monitoring a household over time cannot be limited to observing changes in the occupants of a given dwelling. Such an approach could only be used to monitor sedentary households. But when a couple with children moves in to house B, this does not amount to the creation of a household any more than the couple's departure from house A corresponds to the disappearance of a household. It is impossible to say unequivocally when households are created or cease to exist. Is a new household created when a young man leaves his parents' home and moves into his girlfriend's apartment? Similarly, does a household cease to exist when two partners separate, even if they continue to live under the same roof? This raises the question of whose household we follow. A "household" defined in terms of physical location is inadequate for describing the history of a family group.

This reality, which inevitably becomes apparent when adopting a longitudinal perspective, prompted us to question traditional statistical units of analysis and challenge the conventional concepts used to identify the visible framework of social morphology. The life event history perspective we adopted gave us further cause to question the traditional markers of the structure. Each individual life-course needs to be put into context. While there may be a series of households in a person's life, relationships – especially family relationships – with people who do not, or no longer, belong to the person's current household, may remain unchanged. To capture this reality accurately, we are proposing the new concept of "entourage", which avoids having to choose between the household and the family because it encompasses both the domestic group and the key people in a person's family network. How these key people are to be identified is still under discussion. It may be up to the individual respondent to identify them, as was done in the *Proches et parents* survey; another way might be to systematically include parents, children and partners, as was our approach.

There are two aspects to the operationality of the principles introduced above: the data and the analysis. If we wish to follow a person's entourage as defined above and identify the successive roles that he/she has held, and the successive households he/she has belonged to, which data will we need?

To assess an individual's changing role, defined in terms of fundamental demographic variables, there is no need to collect additional data if we already have information about all the conjugal unions and reproductive events. The model is highly simplified in this initial outline; if we were to make it more complex, we might want to gather data about the location over time of children and parents (relationships of direct descent) when the respondent does not live with either his/her parents or children. As we can see, this additional information does not, in principle, represent an insurmountable obstacle in terms of data collection.

In addition to changes in the individual's position, it is important to identify the different types of co-residence, i.e. the nature of the daily interactions over the individual's life course; in other words, the composition of the successive households to which the individual had belonged. This was done in the *Peuplement et dépeuplement de Paris* survey.

This type of analysis would make it possible to interpret individual behaviour, currently considered independently of the family and social context. The aim is, firstly, to incorporate inter-generational factors into the analysis of residential and occupational (and even demographic) behaviours, and, secondly, to identify the interactions that develop between individuals and their entourage.

This would make it possible to study decisions about residential mobility in relation to the location of various family members. For instance, does moving to Paris mean being farther from family or closer to them? Similarly, we could attempt to determine whether there was a regular pattern between family relationships and geographical location over the life course – e.g. an individual first moves out of home to a location close to their parents, then moves farther away after forming a union, and then moves closer again when they have children, or when their parents grow old. Regarding interactions between the individual histories of peers, the most salient example is that of the relocations that occur when a union is dissolved, especially in cases where there are children.

In conclusion, if we wish to capture the complexity of an individual's relationships with his/her family and entourage, we believe it is important to reach beyond the restrictive statistical framework of the family group within the household and introduce the time component into the analysis of the individual's constellation of relationships in order to better understand the meaning of family, residential and social histories. The aim of this new conceptual tool is to reinterpret historical and sociological developments in family structures by going beyond an instrumental view of interactions between relatives. In this light, families would no longer be perceived in terms of assistance given or received or the frequency of contact observed at a given point in time, but in terms of bonds that have developed over time and how these are reflected in space, both geographical and social.

References

Audirac, P. A. (1985). Les personnes âgées, de la vie de famille à l'isolement. *Économie et statistiques*.

Bonvalet, C., Maison, D., Le Bras, H., & Charles, L. (1993). Proches et parents. *Population, 48*(1), 83–110.

Bourdieu, P. (1993). À propos de la famille comme catégorie réalisée. *Actes de la recherche en sciences sociales*, 100.

Caplow, T., Bart, H., & Chadwick, B. (1982). *Middletown families. Fifty years of change and continuity*. Minneapolis: University of Minnesota Press.

Courgeau, D. (1972). Les réseaux de relations entre personnes. Étude d'un milieu rural. *Population, 27*(4–5), 641–683.

Courgeau, D. (1975). Les réseaux de relations entre personnes. Études dans un milieu urbain. *Population, 30*(2), 271–283.
Courgeau, D., & Lelièvre, E. (1989). *Analyse démographique des biographies*. Paris: INED, coll. "Manuels".
de Saboulin, M. (1984). The family structure and households in France. Réunion franco-allemande, Trêves.
de Saboulin, M. (1986). Households and family characteristics in the population census of France. In *Conference of European Statistics (ONU)* (Working Paper), Geneva.
de Singly, F. (1993) *Comment définir la famille contemporaine*. Solidarité Santé, Études statistiques du ministère des Affaires sociales et de l'Intégration, 4.
Desrosières, A. (1993). *La politique des grands nombres, histoire de la raison statistique*. Paris: Éditions La Découverte.
Duncan, G., & Morgan, J. (Eds.). (1983). *Five thousand American families: Patterns of economy progress*. Ann Arbor: Institute for Social Research, University of Michigan.
Durr, J.-M. (1991). *Nuptialité et structures des ménages*. Paris: INED, coll. Congrès et colloques, 7.
Flandrin, J.-L. (1976). *Familles, parenté, maison, sexualité dans l'ancienne société*. Paris: Hachette, coll. "Le temps et les hommes".
Gokalp, C. (1978). Le réseau familial". *Population, 33*(6), 1077–1094.
Henry, L. (1972). *Démographie, analyse et modèles*. Paris: Larousse (republished 1984, INED).
Kuijsten, A., & Vossen, A. (1988). Introduction. In N. Keilman, A. Kuijsten, & A. Vossen (Eds.), *Modelling household formation and dissolution*. Oxford: Oxford University Press.
Laslett, P. (1972). *Household and family in past time* (623 p.). Cambridge: Cambridge University Press.
Le Bras H. (1979). *L'Enfant et la famille dans les pays de l'OCDE: analyse démographique*. OCDE, Centre pour la recherche et l'innovation dans l'enseignement.
Le Faucheur, N. (1988). Les familles monoparentales en questions. *Dialogue, 101*, 28–44.
Lefranc, C. (1995). Ménages et familles : constructions statistiques et réalités nationales; une comparaison entre l'Allemagne, la France et la Grande Bretagne. *Revue des affaires sociales*, N°4.
Le Play, F. (1871). *L'organisation de la famille selon le vrai modèle signalé par l'histoire de toutes les races et de tous les temps*. Paris: Tequi.
Le Play, F. (1901). *La réforme sociale en France déduite de l'observation comparée des peuples européens, tome I: La religion, la propriété, la famille*. Tours: Maison Alfred Mame.
Mermet, J.-C. (1988). Pratiques sociales de l'habitat et dynamiques de la divortialité. In C. Bonvalet & P. Merlin (Eds.), *Transformations de la famille et habitat*. Paris: INED, DREIF, IDEF, coll "Travaux et Documents", 120.
Parsons, T., & Bales, R. F. (1955). *Family, socialization and family patterns*. Glencoe: The Free Press.
Prioux, F. (1990). *La Famille dans les pays développés: permanence et changements*. In F. Prioux (Eds.), Congrès et Colloques, Paris, INED, Recensement de la population de 1990, Ménages – Familles, résultats du sondage au quart.
Ryder, N.-B. (1985). Recent developments in the formal demography of the family. In *International population conférence*, Florence (Vol. 3, pp. 207–220). Liège: IUSSP.
Segalen, M. (1993). *Sociologie de la famille*. Paris: Armand Colin.
Théry, I. (1991). Trouver le mot juste. Langage et parenté dans les recompositions familiales après divorce. In M. Segalen (Ed.), *Jeux de famille*. Paris: CNRS Éditions.
Villac, M. (1991). Les structures familiales se transforment profondément. *Économie et statistiques*, 152.
Young, M., & Willmott, P. (1957). *Family and kinship in East London*. London: Routledge and Kegan Paul.

Chapter 4
Between Socially-Instituted Parental Relationships and Elective Ones: A Retrospective Analysis of Parent Figures in France from 1930 to 1965

Éva Lelièvre, Géraldine Vivier, and Christine Tichit

At a time when the broad diversity of family structures, newly emerging or otherwise, is reshaping the very notion of parenthood, this study aims to place current research and debate in a more long-term perspective by revisiting the parental and educational universe of the cohorts born between 1930 and 1950. In addition to biological parents, adoptive parents and step-parents, this paper also focuses on individuals mentioned by respondents as having played a parental role when they were children, and on their descriptions of the circumstances and histories of their childhoods. We propose a dual change of perspective. First, the parental relationship is not broached from the viewpoint of the adults who played a parental role but from that of the children, now adults. Second, it is not restricted to biological or socially-instituted parents. While earlier studies examined elective parental relationships through adoption (Fine 1998), we would like to expand this by analysing original material that provides a "practical" view of the relationship.

The *Biographies et entourage* survey retraced the family, residential and occupational trajectories of 2830 individuals aged between 50 and 70 in the Paris region, and extended the field of observation to close friends and relatives. In this way the survey was able to locate individuals within their family group, and more broadly, in their families' sphere of influence, in order to understand the role of the family network in their life course and see how it evolved over time (Lelièvre and Vivier

This article first appeared in the journal *Population*, *English Edition*, (63) 2, pp. 209–238.

É. Lelièvre (✉) • G. Vivier
Institut national d'études démographiques (INED), Paris, France
e-mail: eva@ined.fr

C. Tichit
UR 1303 Alimentation et sciences sociales (ALISS), Institut national de recherches agronomiques (INRA), Paris, France

C. Bonvalet, É. Lelièvre (eds.), *Family Beyond Household and Kin*,
INED Population Studies 6, DOI 10.1007/978-3-319-24684-0_4

2001). The data collected enable us to reconstruct the respondents' situations at each moment in their history, not just within their own trajectories but also with respect to their close contact circle, the family circle in particular,[1] and to follow their progress.

When applied to a specific segment of this network, namely the persons and institutions who comprised the parental and educational universe of the cohorts born between 1930 and 1950, analysis of this data of dynamic networks reveals that an extraordinary diversity of parental and educational entities took charge of these cohorts, in addition to their biological parents. Our research identifies the circumstances under which a parental function was exercised and the roles that parent figures incarnated in association – or in competition – with the biological parents. We endeavour to go beyond the family background to understand the social and historic context in which these cohorts grew up, and the framework in which these relationships were constructed. Lastly, by analysing respondents' descriptions of their parent figures, we attempt to identify the functions attributed to these "other parents" in order to examine the distribution of roles between the adults who made up the parental and educational universe of these cohorts, and to situate the "elective parents" who replaced or complemented the biological or socially-instituted parents.

In fact, over and above the empirical results we present here, this study raises questions of history, anthropology, sociology of the family and demography, paving the way for important methodological discussions. The results of our research into the little-known familial and extra-familial resources that were mobilized by the children and/or their families for educational purposes from the 1930s to the mid 1960s contribute to current debate and research on parenting.

4.1 The Issue of Parenthood in the *Biographies et entourage* Survey

In the 2001 survey carried out by INED on 2830 inhabitants of Ile-de-France (Paris region), the parental universe included a range of figures: the biological parents, if applicable, the adoptive parents, the mother or father's partner with whom the respondent had lived, along with any other person or persons identified by the respondent as playing a parental role. Box 4.1 provides details on the data collected on these various figures.

This fairly broad definition explains the concept of "parental universe" used here, which is better suited to the diversity of people who played a parenting role at a given time, whether simultaneously or successively. This is not a natural definition in societies where the notion of parenthood is strongly connected to the unique and exclusive roles of the mother and father (Fine 2001). We will therefore begin by

[1] The close contact circle, as defined for data collection, included the respondent's blood relatives and relatives by marriage, plus all persons with whom the respondent had lived as well as other persons they freely referred to as having played a key role in their lives.

explaining how this concept took shape at the questionnaire design stage and how we analysed the qualitative and quantitative data collected in this survey.

Box 4.1: Summary of Data from the *Biographies et entourage* Survey (INED 2001) Used to Analyse the Parental Universe
The parental circle that we investigated included:

- biological fathers and mothers, if applicable,
- adoptive fathers and mothers,
- partners of the father and/or mother (if they lived with the respondent),
- other persons who played a parental role, or a so-called "parent figure".

Data relating to parent figures (see further details in the Appendix) included:

- the person's individual characteristics: sex, main events in his/her conjugal and family life (unions, separations, children, etc.), main activity (occupation, status, economic sector);
- the connection between that person and the respondent: type of relationship (uncle, sister, neighbour, teacher, etc.), when the relationship began and the period during which that person was influential, their place of residence in relation to the respondent (co-resident, same *commune* or neighbouring *commune*, elsewhere) at the time this person was influential, and current residence, frequency of contacts at the time and at present, role played by this person and the circumstances under which s/he played a parental role: "Why was this person important? How did he/she play a parental role for you?".

The residential trajectories of respondents indicated for each period:

- the type of housing (individual or collective) the respondent lived in;
- all the persons with whom s/he lived (father, mother, father or mother's spouse, brother, sister, grandfather, grandmother, non-relative, etc.).

4.1.1 From "Father" and "Mother" to the "Parental Universe": The Origins of the Questionnaire

The first versions of the *Biographies et entourage* questionnaire merely asked the parents' date of birth and, if applicable, date of death, without defining the word "parent" in any way, but implicitly assumed the unique and unambiguous meaning of what was asked. From the outset, however, this framework was found to be unsuitable and too narrow because several parents or "pairs" of parents emerged, such as adoptive parents following the death of deported biological parents, for instance. No one parent appeared to be more important or legitimate than the other, and therefore no selection could be relevant or acceptable, especially in the framework of a biographical approach that intended to explore the influence of the respondents' close family circle throughout their life course.

In the following test we broadened the scope of the question to "all persons who had a parental role" which enabled us to include adoptive parents and confirmed the existence of additional and/or alternative figures to the biological parents. At this stage, 37 respondents out of a total of 116 mentioned the existence of at least one person who played a parental role in their lives. A total of 59 persons were referred to in this way. Nevertheless, this approach also revealed the complexities that lay behind the notion of "parent", from established framework to personal reality and individual perception. Parents' partners (i.e. step-parents) who might be thought to belong to this category, were not necessarily identified by respondents as having "played a parental role", even when they lived together for many years. Conversely, other unexpected figures were mentioned, whether or not they had lived with the respondent. In short, the test revealed that certain socially-instituted parent figures were not necessarily viewed as such by respondents, whereas other persons not usually perceived as having these roles were included in the parental universe. This introduced a notion of choice in the identification of a parental relationship, which is usually instituted and not chosen (at least from the child's viewpoint).

Clearly, from the respondents' viewpoint, a daily presence in the home was not sufficient[2] to confer a parental role upon a co-resident adult, or for the adult to be accepted as a parent figure, while individuals who did not co-reside, were not disqualified from assuming this role. This disconnection between co-residence, the "nurturing" function and the parent figure led us to look in greater detail at the ties of affinity that are probably implicit in recognizing or attributing a parental function and a parental relationship.

In this respect, while not producing statistically reliable data, this same test, which systematically explored the affective ties between the respondent and his/her close family circle,[3] produced some interesting results. Only 4 respondents out of the 37 who referred to a person having played a parental role, reported that they were not "close" to that person, while 22 respondents out of 116 reported, in the same precise terms, that they were not "close" to their biological father and/or mother. A juxtaposition of these observations would suggest that while feeling close to one's biological parents – rarely contested – is not, paradoxically, self-evident, conversely, appointing a parent figure presupposes a certain quality of relationship and affection (even if not automatic). This comparison of socially-instituted parents and elective parents recalls the purely elective relational model analysed by Sabine Chalvon-Demersay in her study of television films broadcast in France in 1995. The author demonstrated that all the screenplays dealt with "the relational upheavals that have occurred in our society over the past 30 years, and the cognitive resources

[2] At the time of the survey, 40 years later.

[3] The question we asked systematically for brothers, sisters, biological parents, persons who played a parental role and children, was "were you close?" (or "were you close before he/she died?"), the only possible reply being "yes" or "no".

available to manage the consequences and explore the implications of an ideal 'world of elective relationships' in which all relationships are based on ties of affection, freely consented and not institutional or constraining" (Chalvon-Demersay 1996, pp. 82–83). In our very different context of cohorts born between 1930 and 1950, our exploration of respondents' parental universes led us to include parent figures who were recognized as such on the basis of both affinity and choice.

Faced with the diversity of situations we found in the tests and the unexpected complexity behind the notion of "parent", the final version of the questionnaire included different combinations of figures who were biologically or socially instituted in parental functions, along with more elective figures. First, biological parents were systematically included, along with adoptive parents and parents' partners (when they had lived with the respondents). Then we explored any other persons identified by respondents as "having played the role of a parent".[4] In further tests, data collected from a large-scale survey confirmed the relevance of this category. Far from causing any surprise or ambiguity among respondents who had just related in detail the trajectories of their biological parents, or of their adoptive and/or step-parents, these parent figures were mentioned (as we shall see) by a non-negligible proportion of individuals.

Finally we should stress that the data concerning these parent figures and the roles they played were provided by the respondents looking back over their life course since childhood. This question thus provided information on the way in which respondents, now on the brink of old age, perceived their childhoods and the adults who took a part in their education.

4.1.2 *Frequency of References to Alternative or Additional Parent Figures*

The frequency with which the various members of the parental and educational universe, alongside or in place of biological parents, were cited as being influential before age 15,[5] revealed their importance. A total of 1008 persons were cited, whether adoptive parents, spouses of parents or non-family parent figures.

While few respondents lived with adoptive parents, family universes are more often reshaped by the repartnering of a parent, with the presence of a stepmother being relatively more frequent. A striking number of respondents mentioned a

[4] For convenience, we shall call parent figures those persons designated in a parental role but not necessarily biologically or even socially instituted as parents.

[5] We should stress that for reasons of consistency we concentrated on the parental universe of respondents between the ages of 0–14 years, up to the end of the compulsory school age in France for those cohorts. Beyond that age, other processes intervened, particularly in respondents' occupational trajectories, since many went into apprenticeships and became fairly autonomous at a fairly early age following their entry into the workforce.

Table 4.1 Percentage of respondents who mentioned persons in their parental and educational universe other than their biological parents before age 15

Persons who played a parental role (called parent figures)	Number of respondents concerned	%
Adoptive parents	28	1.0
Father's spouses	103	3.6
Mother's spouses	50	1.8
Total	585	21.0

Note: Certain step-parents or adoptive parents already mentioned may also have been cited as playing a parental role
Source: *Biographies et entourage* survey (INED 2001)

person who played a parental role for them before age 15: more than one fifth referred to at least one such parent figure (Table 4.1).

We should add that no typical profile emerged from the socio-demographic characteristics of respondents who designated a parent figure. Although men and women did not describe parent figures in the same terms or attribute the same functions to them (as will be detailed later), they appeared in the children's universe independently of the respondent's sex.

Similarly – and paradoxically one might say – an only-child was more likely to mention a parent figure than a respondent with brothers and sisters, though the differences remain small. The number of brothers and sisters was not a determining factor and neither was social background or place of birth.

Two-thirds of respondents concerned mentioned having one parent figure and 60 % of those who mentioned several figures usually referred to couples. Individuals born before the war mentioned slightly more parent figures than others, especially in the specific context of the war, but few mentioned more than two people, and a total of 803 individuals were identified as "having played a parental role" in the respondents' childhood and adolescence.

Before analysing how all these parental figures combined to make up the respondents' parental and educational universe, we will first look more closely at these more elective parents who complemented or replaced the biological or socially-instituted parents. Who were these parent figures? What ties did they have with the respondents? In what framework did they exercise their parental function?

4.2 Who Were the Parent Figures?

They are mostly female (67 % women and 33 % men) and are usually related to the respondent (Tables 4.2 and 4.3). Nevertheless they include a broad range of relationships (28 different ones) covering a span of three generations: 63 % were from the grandparents', or occasionally the great-grandparents', generation; 27 % were from the parents' generation: aunts and uncles, etc., and 10 % were from the same generation as the respondents: brothers, sisters, cousins, etc.

Table 4.2 Distribution of parent figures according to their relationship with respondents

Relationship		Percentage	Number
Family	Grandparent	60	676 (84 %)
	Uncle or aunt	27	
	Brother or sister	8	
	Other relative	6	
	Total	*100*	
Outside the family	Household employee, childminder	37	127 (16 %)
	Foster family	20	
	Godfather or godmother	16	
	Neighbour or friend	6	
	Other non-related person	22	
	Total	*100*	
All persons who played a parental role			803 (100 %)

Coverage: Individuals mentioned by respondents as having played a parental role in their childhood
Source: *Biographies et entourage* survey (INED 2001)

Table 4.3 Distribution of parent figures by sex and relationship with respondents (%)

Relationship with respondent		Number	Breakdown by sex	
			Men	Women
Family	Grandparents	51	30	70
	Uncle or aunt	20	42	58
	Brother or sister	8	36	64
	Other relative	5	27	73
Outside the family	Contractual relationship with parents	7	11	89
	Other non-related figure	9	40	60
Total %		*100*	*33*	*67*
Number of respondents		803	259	544

Coverage: Individuals mentioned by respondents as having played a parental role in their childhood
Source: *Biographies et entourage* survey (INED 2001)

At a time when the "new role" of grandparents and their closer involvement with grandchildren is taking the limelight (Attias-Donfut et al. 2002), it is important to stress that in 50 % of cases these alternative or supplementary parents are a grandmother or grandfather. Grandparents were very active, comprising the majority of the couples mentioned as parent figures, and hence frequently a part of the parental and educational universe of these respondents born between 1930 and 1950. Uncles and aunts were the second most frequently mentioned category of relatives, followed by older brothers and sisters (Table 4.2). "Other relatives" included people from the grandparents' generation (great-uncles and great-aunts) as well as those of the respondents' generation (cousins).

Even more unexpectedly, 16 % of the parent figures are not blood relatives of the respondents, which reinforces the elective dimension of the designated parent figure. First and foremost were persons who had a contractual relationship with the parents (childminder, household employee). Then came the foster families and godparents.[6] The female figure of the nursemaid/childminder dominates. This extra-familial parental universe was, however, extremely diversified and included a broad range of persons in the child's daily life (neighbours, network of friends, teachers, etc.) or people they met under the exceptional circumstances in which these generations of children grew up.

More than three-quarters of respondents (79 %) mentioned one parent figure, usually a woman and generally the grandmother. Male respondents were more likely to mention male figures and often referred to them as one part of a "parenting couple" rather than as separate individuals. Childminders and household employees were invariably female (Table 4.3). We will below look in greater detail at the gender affinities between the respondents and their reported parent figures.

In addition to the relationships between respondents and their parent figures, the personal trajectories of these surrogate parents are revealing. Their own family situations were such that they had the necessary free time to play a parental role. Grandparents had ceased to raise their own children when they were active in respondents' lives and most of the other relatives in parental roles did not have children (or not yet). This was the case for 40 % of the uncles and aunts and 80 % of the older brothers and sisters who were still very young when they took on a parental role for respondents. Several respondents[7] stressed the unmarried status of their parent figures or the fact that they were childless.

> Referring to an aunt: "She was like a second mother to me. She never had any children, so she loved me and my brother like her own."
>
> On the subject of a godmother who was a primary school teacher, "She was a spinster, and she took me with her on holiday, made me do my homework and paid for special tuition, such as piano lessons."

These extracts suggest that not only were educational tasks distributed amongst available adults, but that these adults had a personal involvement with their charges, or even some emotional need directly related to the absence of a child. This raises questions about the reciprocal nature of the relationship and the gratitude that it implies. Respondents designated these persons as having played a parental role for them, but these individuals also devoted themselves to that role and to the relationship.

[6] It is striking that godparents, whether related or not, only represented 6 % of all the parent figures mentioned. In this study we placed related godfather or godmother in their relevant category of relative. As a result "godparents" only includes non-related persons (a mere 2.5 %).

[7] The quotations are from replies to the open-ended questions in the questionnaire and recorded *verbatim* in the files.

4.2.1 *When Did They Play a Parental Role and in What Circumstances?*

Most parent figures, especially those who belonged to the family circle, assumed their roles in the respondents' early childhood if not at their birth (Table 4.4). That was especially true of grandparents, 80 % of whom played a key role before respondents reached 6 years of age.

The starting point at which the non-related persons became influential was more variable, with contractual figures such as childminders and household employees mostly appearing early in respondents' childhoods, and other non-related persons usually becoming influential around age 6, although they are not necessarily associated with a specific age.

On average, respondents were 6 years old when they first came under the influence of parent figures and this influence often lasted beyond childhood and after age 15 for half the persons mentioned, or even a lifetime for 6 %.

Cohabitation during all or part of the period of influence often affected the relationship. Some 65 % of parent figures lived with the respondents, and only friends, godparents and neighbours did not cohabit, although 44 % lived close by (Lelièvre et al. 2005).

While sharing day-to-day life under the same roof fostered parental influence (Gollac 2003), it did not automatically lead to a parental relationship, since one third of the figures mentioned did not cohabit with the respondent. Conversely, other adults (related or otherwise) sometimes lived with respondents for several years without ever being designated as a parent figure.

Table 4.4 Respondents' age at start of parent figures' period of influence, by type of relationship (%)

Relationship	From birth	Ages 1–5	Ages 6–9	Age 10+	Total	*Number*
Family	45	27	19	8	100	*676*
Grandparent	51	28	16	4	100	*403*
Uncle, aunt	35	29	23	11	100	*165*
Brother, sister	43	10	26	21	100	*52*
Other relative	32	34	18	13	100	*56*
Outside the family	29	24	29	16	100	*127*
Childminder	39	33	20	7	100	*54*
Other non-relative	22	18	37	23	100	*73*

Coverage: Individuals mentioned by respondents as having played a parental role in their childhood

Interpretation: 45 % of parent figures exercised "a key influence" from respondent's birth and 8 % from age 10

Source: *Biographies et entourage* survey (INED 2001)

4.3 Configurations of the Parental Universe between 0 and 14 Years

We will now look at the composition of the parental universe of respondents aged between 0 and 14 years. To do so, we reconstructed each respondent's parental universe by taking into account the biological father and mother if they were known and were alive during the period in question, the father's or mother's spouse(s) if they co-resided with the respondent, adoptive parents and parent figures who exerted an influence before age 15.

The parental configurations describe the composition of the probable (or actual) parental and educational universes of the respondents and make no assumptions regarding the role each figure actually played. Moreover, it was possible for the persons cited to be present in the configuration simultaneously or successively between ages 0 and 14.

We obtained more precise dating for periods of presence or absence of biological parents by analysing the respondents' residential trajectory and the composition of their households, taking into account periods spent in an institution, such as a boarding school, or in other households (related or otherwise) where respondents may have been placed.

The variety of situations we found was quite striking. The majority configuration (69.8 %) was the one in which the two biological parents made up the exclusive parental universe (at least in theory[8]), but quite frequently (in 18.6 % of cases) a third external person supplemented the two parents. Nearly one respondent in four grew up in a universe where the father, mother or both biological parents were not the only members of the parental universe (Table 4.5).

Second, we observed that the mother was, by far, the figure most present for respondents. Only 4.2 % lost their mothers before age 15 compared with 9 % who lost their fathers by the same age. This imbalance reveals the impact of the war on the parental universe of these cohorts. A total of 12 % of respondents had lost one or both of their biological parents by age 15.

A detailed examination of the 585 configurations in which alternative parent figures appeared – or, to be precise, persons identified by respondents as playing a parental role before they reached age 15 (Table 4.5, last columns) – revealed that in most cases the parent figures were supplemental to biological parents who were alive even if not present on a daily basis. However, more than 20 % of respondents with a parent figure in their parental universe, were orphaned before age 15.

In relative terms, 37.5 % of respondents who had lost either their father and/or their mother before age 15[9] mentioned having at least one parent figure. These alternative figures are thus over-represented in the event of a parent's death. However,

[8] At this stage, biological parents are included in the configuration if they are alive throughout the observation period, from 0 to 14 years, independently of their effective presence (co-residence) with the respondent.

[9] Or 12 % of total respondents.

Table 4.5 Configurations of respondents' potential parental universes before age 15 by presence of parent figures

Composition of the parental universe		All respondents		Those reporting a parent figure	
	Number	%		Number	%
Mother + father alive	**1975**	**69.79**			
+ one parent figure	429	15.16		429	
+ one of parents' spouses[a]	54	1.91	88.0	4[b]	79.3
+ a parent figure and one of parents' spouses	24	0.85		24	
+ at least two other people: parent figure/adoptive parent or one of parents' spouses	10	0.35		6	
Mother alive	**130**	**4.59**			
+ one parent figure	49	1.73		49	
+ the mother's spouse	25	0.88	7.8		10.8
+ a parent figure + mother's spouse	13	0.46		13	
+ an adoptive parent	3	0.11		1	
Father alive	**27**	**0.95**			
+ one parent figure	29	1.02		29	
+ father's spouse	19	0.67	3.0	5	7.3
+ a parent figure + father's spouse	9	0.32		9	
+ an adoptive parent	1	0.04			
Father and mother dead or unknown	**33**	**1.17**	1.2	15	2.6
Total	2830	100.0	100.0	585	100.0

[a]Possibly also designated as a parent figure
[b]Parent's spouse designated as a parent figure
Source: *Biographies et entourage* survey (INED 2001)

among the 88 % in the sample with both parents, 18.5 % mentioned an additional person in a parental role. So over and above a "substitution" or "compensation" effect, we see the existence of third parties "appended" to the traditional parent couple.

4.3.1 Cohabitation with Biological Parents

Taking account of respondents' cohabitation with their father and mother enabled us to refine our analysis by integrating breaks in co-residence with biological parents lasting at least 1 year, for whatever reason: death, marital breakdown, geographical separation due to war, parents' work, respondents' schooling, etc. (Lelièvre and Vivier 2006).

Table 4.6 Configurations of respondents' actual parental universes before age 15

Composition	Number	%	Cum.%
Mother + biological father in uninterrupted co-residence	1384	48.9	
+ parent figure	142	5.0	53.9
Mother's uninterrupted co-residence	389	13.7	
+ parent figure	96	3.4	
+ mother's spouse	48	1.7	
+ parent figure + mother's spouse	6	0.2	19.0
Father's uninterrupted co-residence	37	1.3	
+ parent figure	20	0.7	
+ father's spouse	9	0.3	
+ parent figure + father's spouse	3	0.1	2.4
No biological parent or other in uninterrupted co-residence	324	11.5	
No biological parent in uninterrupted co-residence but:			
One parent figure in uninterrupted co-residence	274	9.7	
Parent figure + other person in uninterrupted co-residence	44	1.5	
Other person in uninterrupted co-residence (a parent's spouse, adoptive parent)	54	1.9	24.6
Total	2830	100.0	100.0

Source: *Biographies et entourage* survey (INED 2001)

Thus when we take into account the actual presence of parents in the household (Table 4.6), we see that only 54 % of respondents actually grew up with both their biological parents from age 0 to 14 without an interruption of more than 1 year, and that in 9 % of cases, the parents' presence did not exclude the influence of another person. Last, only 48.9 % of respondents lived in the type of configuration in which the biological father or mother made up the sole, exclusive, parent couple in continuous co-residence with the respondent.

Conversely, a remarkably large proportion of respondents (46 %) did not live continually with their two parents up to age 15 (and in come cases never lived with them) because cohabitation was interrupted with the mother or the father, or with both parents, before that age:

- 21.5 % of respondents cohabited continuously with one of their biological parents. In the majority of cases, the father was absent from the household: 19 % of respondents lived at least 1 year with their mother[10] but without their father. The reverse (father present, mother absent) was rare and concerned only 2.5 % of respondents.
- 24.6 % spent at least 1 year without their father *and* 1 year without their mother on a daily basis before age 15. In the vast majority of cases, the father and mother were absent simultaneously (at least some of the time). Only seven individuals had never experienced the simultaneous absence of both parents, since their parents alternated their periods of absence.

[10] Alone or otherwise.

Taking all the situations together, 27 % of respondents spent at least 1 year without their mothers and 44 % without their fathers.[11]

The modal duration of separation for respondents who had experienced simultaneous interruption of co-residence with both parents (the case for 689 respondents) was 1 year,[12] but just over half of respondents had in fact spent between 1 and 4 years without their parents.

4.3.2 *Time Spent in Boarding Schools, Institutions and with Third Parties*

Persons living in an institution for at least 1 year before age 15, necessarily ceased to live with their two parents on a daily basis, and 336 (or 12 %) out of the total 2830 respondents were in this situation. Three-quarters of them were at boarding school but there were also periods in orphanages, sanatoriums, preventive health institutions and other medical structures, detention/correction centres, hostels for refugees or emergency shelters.

Half of those who ceased to reside with both parents for at least 1 year (Table 4.7) were in boarding school. Periods in boarding schools were not just the result of an educational choice or the absence of a suitable local school. They often coincided with other events such as parents' separation, migration etc. that affected family life

Table 4.7 Time spent in an institution and the parental universe of children whose co-residence with both parents was interrupted before age 15

Type of parental universe	Number	%
Time spent in an institution	**336**	**48.8**
Father and mother continuously absent and at least one other person in parental universe	127	18.4
Father and mother continuously absent and no other person in parental universe	209	30.3
No time spent in an institution	**353**	**51.2**
Father and mother continuously absent and at least one other person in parental universe	238	34.5
Father and mother continuously absent and no other person in parental universe	115	16.7
Total	**689**	**100.0**

Coverage: Respondents who did not live continuously with their two biological parents before age 15
Source: *Biographies et entourage* survey (INED 2001)

[11] These respondents lived on average 11.46 years with their mother and 8.26 years with their father. The difference is not significant, however.

[12] The modal duration is the most frequent duration, i.e. 17 % of respondents concerned.

Table 4.8 Relationship with the reference person in the household where respondent was placed before age 15

Relationship with respondent	Number	%
Grandfather and/or grandmother	160	44.7
Uncle and/or aunt	63	17.6
Foster family	58	16.2
Adopted parents	28	7.8
Brother and/or sister	12	3.3
Other relative (cousins, father's or mother's spouse etc.)	16	4.5
Friends	6	1.7
Godfather/godmother[a]	4	1.1
Other non-related persons	11	3.1
Total	358	100.0

[a]The number of godparents could be underestimated as they could also be designated by another relationship (uncle and aunt for instance)
Coverage: Respondents who lived for at least 1 year before age 15 in a household other than that of one or both of their parents
Source: *Biographies et entourage* survey (INED 2001)

(Lelièvre et al. 2005). Boarding school may have been perceived by parents as a means to take charge of the children at a difficult time in their life course.

Periods in boarding school were half as frequent for those who mentioned at least one person in the parental universe other than their biological father and mother: 34.8 % went to boarding school compared with 65.2 % of those who had no other person in the parental universe between ages 0 and 14.

Apart from boarding school, another form of separation with parents consisted of placing children with third parties[13] thereby mobilizing different resources and educational figures. Half the children who were separated from both parents simultaneously before age 15 were in the care of a third party.[14] The identification of the "resource persons" who took charge of these children again reveals the potentialities of blood ties: nearly half the children were sent to live with their grandparents (for at least 1 year) who thus constituted the primary source of backup childcare (Table 4.8). Remember that grandparents are also the people most often mentioned by respondents as having played a parental role before age 15, frequently in the context of co-residence. After grandparents came uncles and aunts and, less frequently, other family members, brothers and sisters, cousins, etc.

Last, children were not only fostered out to informal care, but also officially to foster families or adoptive parents, who in some cases were related to the respondents.

[13] And, much more rarely, into apprenticeships or into very early marriages.

[14] Being placed in a boarding school and with a third party were not mutually exclusive.

4.3.3 Historical and Family Contexts: From War to Working Mothers

The childhoods of these cohorts (1930–1950) were marked by major social and political events, such as the French *Front populaire*, World War II and reconstruction, rural exodus, all of which affected children's daily lives. Events cited include the first children's holiday camps, the trauma of the civilian exodus after the German invasion and the war-time evacuation of children, (see for example, Downs 2002). While the context in which the parent figures were mentioned varied a great deal in this period (1930–1965), our data shows no significant difference in the propensity to cite a parent figure according to the context, including the war years (1939–1945) which one might suppose to be an important period for parent figures. Certain figures were typical of the war era, namely the so-called "other non-related persons" (neither godparents, nor neighbours, nor domestic servants) who were mostly mentioned during this period, alongside foster families. For children who had lost parents in the war or whose families were destroyed or dispersed, the impact of the war inevitably continued into peace time. Most foster families[15] are mentioned by "war orphans" after the war. Strikingly, many of the statements about parent figures during the war did not reveal a traumatic vision of the period, but referred to memories of daily life that were often quite happy. This viewpoint contrasts with today's descriptions of the period, dominated by collective memory and by government child protection policies that have crystallized memories of a traumatized war generation (Downs 2005). While war played a role in the emergence of certain family configurations, it does not alone explain the frequency and diversity of the parent figures that were mentioned. The majority of these parent figures exerted an influence outside the war period, in the 1930s for one quarter of them, and after the war for the majority (44 %).[16]

Before the war, the majority of persons in parental roles were the grandparents (59 %); but this was no longer the case in 1940 (below 50 %). Only uncles and aunts were mentioned regularly over the whole period. After the war and in the 1950s, brothers and sisters appeared more frequently, as did people from outside the family such as friends, whose role was increasing, (especially parents' friends), and neighbours. This shift in the profile of parent figures reflects the changes in the family support network taking place in a context of the rural exodus, rapid urbanization and the housing crisis that characterized 1950s France. Throughout the period from 1930, female employment, while statistically invisible, was impacting the daily organization of households. As respondents explained, the difficulty of reconciling work and family life justified the need for a third party to take over from parents, especially from unavailable mothers (Lelièvre et al. 2005). Methods used varied

[15] Foster families accounted for 3 % of figures who had played a parental role.

[16] The post-war period cumulated the risk of exposure in terms of number of years (20 years, from 1946 to 1965) and of cohorts (all three cohorts are contemporary to this period).

from leaving children at the grandparents' home on a daily or weekly basis, to the regular presence of a person in the child's home, whether under a contractual agreement (household employee, childminder) or not (grandparents, neighbours, etc.).

4.4 The Role of Parent Figures

Let us now look at the types of functions attributed to these "elective parents" and the way the roles – either complementary or surrogate – are distributed between the adults who made up the parental universe. We will focus in particular on the effects of gender and of the type of relationship between respondent and parent figure. We used Réseau-Lu® software to carry out a textual analysis of the 803 replies to the open-ended question,[17] "Why was this person important? How did he/she play a parental role for you?" to understand how respondents perceived these parent figures and the material and affective role they played in their lives.

4.4.1 What Respondents Said About Their Parent Figures

Generally speaking, respondents answered in three types of narrative registers: the functions register (57 %), some of which relate to the biological parents, the circumstances under which the parental role was exercised, and the personal characteristics of the parent figures in question.

The functions attributed to the parent figures were categorized into four main themes: material tasks (*feed, nurse, meet the needs of, mind, take care of*, etc.) learning, socialization and education (*learning about things, contributing*, etc.), affective and psychological roles (*loving, cosseting, being a role model, admiring*, etc.) and lastly, exercising responsibility and authority (Table 4.9). The terms used by respondents evoke practical, day-to-day parenting. We also observed that the five universal functions of parenthood identified by anthropologists (Goody 1999) which consist of *bearing and begetting* descendants, *endowing* them with birth-status identity (legitimation), *nurturing* them, *training* them and introducing them socially into adulthood (*sponsorship*), all appeared in the corpus at different levels, with functions sometimes taken on by persons or institutions in addition to the biological parents.

[17] The Réseau-Lu® software enabled us to calculate the specificity of the words, to homogenize the corpus by lemmatization, to explore the contextual positioning of the words, to analyse the co-occurrence of themes and to make a cross analysis of key words with the modalities of selected variables (Mogoutov and Vichnevskaia 2006). Our corpus of 803 replies generated 8310 thematic propositions (given in Table 4.9). We then specifically analysed the dominant themes that emerged from the corpus according to the respondent's sex and the parent figures they mentioned.

Table 4.9 The main explanatory registers of the role of parent figures

Register	Themes	Frequency %	Frequency Number	Sub-themes
Functions carried out 57 %	Material role	9 %	732	Material support (help, provide for…)
				Health (illness, hospital, care for…)
				Feed (feed, meals, cake…)
				Look after (look after, watch over…)
				Care (take_care_of, shopping, sleeping, laundry…)
	Development	8 %	666	Early learning (learn_about_things, poetry, humour, culture…)
	Socialization			Leisure (cinema, holidays, outings…)
				Contribution (contribute…)
	Nurturing	6 %	499	(Raise, take_care_of…)
	Welcome	6 %	499	Mobility (coming, going, taking…)
	Support			Making welcome (welcome, put up, foster…)
	Affective role	5 %	455	Love_affection (love, cherish, tenderness, cosseting…)
				Respect (respect, admire, recognition…)
				Role model (reference, model…)
	Relationship and psychological framework	5 %	396	Dialogue (talk, listen, say, share…)
				Psychology (confide, trust, affinity, closeness…)
				Influence
				Advice
	Educational role	4 %	347	Studies (school, mathematics…)
				Education (educate, education…)
	Responsibility, authority	3 %	264	Administrative (guardian, adoption, social services…)
				Responsibility (decision, take_on, in_care…)
				Authority (impose, discipline, obey, fear…)
and compared	Comparison	7 %	618	Comparison of adults (more_than, less_than, better_than…)
	Complement/ Substitution	4 %	295	Replace second_ (2nd_ mummy, 2nd _family, 2nd _father…)
Context 28 %	Space temporality	16 %	1316	Time (years, every_day, often, Thursday…)
				Place (house, Paris, France…)
				War (world_war, exodus…)
	Stages of life	6 %	488	(Child_childhood, throughout _life, first communion, marriage…)
	Parental environment	6 %	532	Accident (death, disappearance, divorce…)
				Work (i.e. the fact that parents worked…)
				Absence (alone, away, miss…)
Description of parent figure 14 %	Personality and status	14 %	1203	Quality (funny, nice, stern, strong, present, cheerful…)
				First name
				Occupation or activity
				Indulgence (mischief, whims, give in, rascal…)
				Nature (rabbit_s, earth, flower_s…)
Total		100 %	8310	

Source: *Biographies et entourage* survey (INED 2001)
Coverage: Statements about individuals mentioned by respondents as having played a parental role in their childhoods
Interpretation: Several registers may occur in a single reply. We identified 8310 thematic clauses grouped in this table under themes and sub-themes. Fifty-seven percent of the lemmatized corpus concerns functions exercised by parent figures, including for instance, the "nurturing" function which appears in 6 % of the corpus

The respondents also supplied contextual elements that placed the event in context and specified the circumstances (historical or family) under which the parental role was exercised. Most indications concerned time and space, i.e. when, with what frequency, on what occasion and place, the parent figure first exercised his/her influence. Respondents thus supplied elements of understanding, *reasons* that explained or legitimized the involvement of a third person and that revealed the absences, constraints and difficulties to which their families were subjected and which led to (or "justified") the involvement of another "parent". Tying in with the functions assumed by parent figures, respondents thus defined the various adults who made up their parental universe using terms of comparison, complementarity or substitution.

Last, respondents provided descriptive elements characterizing the personality or the status (social, occupational) of the parent figure, thus giving clues as to why a parental role was attributed to that individual. These characteristics were related less to context (history or family) than to respondents' personal perceptions. They shed light on the functions of these individuals and on the quality and affective dimension of the relationship.

4.4.2 Who Said What About Whom?

Men and women referred equally to the eight parenting functions, whether with regard to caring, help, assistance, nurturing, responsibility, welcoming or supervising (Table 4.10). However, women specifically mentioned notions of psychological and affective care and functions such as intellectual stimulation, whereas the men, whose descriptions were less detailed overall, referred more to practical and educational functions (especially regarding family members) and often summarized the parental role as one of "replacing" parents without providing any specific details.

Women were also more likely to place the exercise of these functions in context and to describe the parent figures, whereas when men broached these aspects, they referred more to the occupational and social identity of the parent figures (worker, employee, in business, daughter of, brother of) and/or specified the context by pointing out its exceptional nature (alone, father prisoner, world war, absent, travel). Women were more likely to describe the person's temperament (cheerful, open, strict, honest, available, sentimental) or their attributes (pipe, plants), and specify the frequency of the relationship (often, Sunday, Thursday, weekly, always, period, per year) and the place (Paris, Trouville, next door, opposite).

These descriptive nuances seem to reveal gender differences in the perception of practical parenting. Men appear to be more marked by the social status of the parent figure and the context, when this was exceptional, whereas the women remained more attached to the description of the personality and the characteristics of the relationship (nature, frequency, place). This suggests that men tend to look for reasons why a third person should enter their parental universe (exceptional circumstances), whereas women appear to attach more importance to the concrete and

Table 4.10 Summary of main functions by respondent's sex and relationship with parent figures (PF)

Functions	Women's discourse		Men's discourse	
	Related PF	Unrelated PF	Related PF	Unrelated PF
Feed – provide for	Grandmother		Aunt	Godfather, godmother
Take care of	Grandmother, sister	Childminder	Aunt	Childminder
Help	brother, sister	Godfather, godmother	Grandfather	Parents' friend
Nurture	Grandmother	Childminder	Grandmother	Childminder
Educate	Grandmother	Godmother	Grandmother, aunt, sister, uncle	Godfather, godmother
Responsibility	Uncle, brother, sister	Godfather	Grandmother, brother	Foster family
Replace parents	Grandparents, brother, sister	Foster family	Grandparents, brother, sister	Godfather, godmother, foster family
Welcome	Uncle, aunt, brother, sister	Parents' friend	–	Foster family, parents' friend
Supervise		Childminder	–	Employer
Affective and psychological role	Grandmother, aunt, sister	Godmother, foster family, childminder	Sister	Foster family
Recreation/leisure	Grandmother, uncle, brother	Childminder, parents' friend	Sister	Childminder, parents' friend
Early learning	Grandparents, aunt, uncle, brother	Godmother, respondents' and parents' friend	Uncle, sister	–
Context and description: Of the person Of the circumstances	Personality, temperament, place, period, frequency		Occupation, activity, war, period	

Coverage: Statements about the individuals mentioned by respondents as having played a parental role in their childhoods
Interpretation: To feed/provide for is a function mentioned with respect to most parent figures, but for men this function is proportionally more often used in relation to aunts among related parent figures, and to godfathers and godmothers among unrelated parent figures
Source: *Biographies et entourage* survey (INED 2001)

factual description of the third person's presence (practical aspects). These differences in perception are doubtless connected to the respondents' later lives and their current position in relation to the practicalities of parenthood. It would be worthwhile to expand the comparative analysis of siblings' discourse where studies have shown that brothers and sisters describe their biological parents differently (Clément 2009; Langevin 1989).

4.4.3 *Predominantly Affectionate Relationships*

Frequently, and in a wide variety of ways, the descriptions of parent figures from the children's viewpoint broach another important aspect of the relationship, namely affection. The affection that occurs in the construction of a feeling of kinship for instance, in the context of Weber's practical kinship (2003), was not identified among the universal functions of parenthood. Yet affection was frequently mentioned in the children's viewpoints that we collected. Over and above the material and supervisory functions of parenting, most respondents mentioned affection and closeness as a decisive factor in the attribution of a parental role. Respondents expressed the *happiness*[18] of living with a grandmother who loved them more than their mother, they were *grateful* to the person who were devoted to their well-being or who took the trouble to intervene on their behalf. This relationship quality was particularly important in the women's statements, showing the existence of this more affective function. Certain individuals were mentioned only because of the exceptional quality of the relationship.

> On the subject of a grandfather[19] with whom the respondent had "spent his life" up to age 10: "He had a little hose-drawn cart and took me out all day. He showed me all sorts of interesting things and explained them, and he would say 'if you're not the strongest you've got to be the smartest'. Not a day passes when I don't think about him."

More generally, psychological and intellectual aspects, as well as early-learning and leisure activities, mostly described by the female respondents, were also described by the male respondents but in relation to their sisters and uncles. There is a kind of crossed relationship between brothers and sisters from this point of view: elder sisters have a special relationship with their younger brothers and elder brothers have a special relationship with younger sisters.

> On the subject of his elder sister, a teacher, a male respondent explained, "She took more care of my schooling than my parents did, helping me get from the 6th grade to the 3rd grade, and into second grade [secondary school classes]; She took me out, or we relaxed, went to the theatre or on cultural outings and she took me on holiday with her."

But for both men and women, the listening and confiding functions remained more in the female circle of sisters and aunts (Table 4.10).

Finally, this affective aspect was occasionally contrasted with tensions in relationships with parents. One respondent remembered neighbours in the same building "where I stayed frequently when my parents were fighting. They taught me

[18] Quotations in *italics* are verbatim extracts from the corpus.

[19] Quotations in the body of the text are taken from transcripts of replies to the open-ended question, as entered into the computer file.

about family life and were very affectionate." This affective aspect reveals the links between the various adults who made up the parental universe. What is at stake for adults, is exercising the parental role. Were the elective parents in competition with the biological ones or substitutes for them? To what extent were they assigned to their role by the parents themselves?

4.4.4 Distribution of Roles: From Complementary to Surrogate

Distributing parent functions between several persons was not just a practical domestic and family arrangement, carried out in the interest of the child. It also served to maintain social bonds, and to ensure their reciprocity and continuity by means of the relationships it generated between adults. Other societies, especially in Africa and Oceania, are more familiar with the idea that parental functions may be held by a variable number of individuals (Goody 1999; Brady 1976), but multi-parenting has always existed in our societies too (Burguière 1993; Lallemand 2002). Whereas today families are reconstituted after divorce or separation, in the past they were reconstituted after widowhood, since death left countless spouses prematurely widowed and gave the surviving spouse the right, if not the social duty, to remarry. Today reconstituted families, assisted reproductive technologies, same-sex parents and adoption are challenging the fundamental criteria of unicity and exclusivity that dominate representations of paternal and maternal roles (Fine 2001; Lallemand 2002; Ouellette 1998). Given the wide variety of parental configurations also observed in these earlier generations, it would be interesting to learn more about the interplay between the different complementary and surrogate parent figures.

The distribution of tasks was often the result of an agreement between adults and organized in a complementary manner, as demonstrated in these comments about an aunt:

> She was there when I was born. My mother and aunt were so close that I can't distinguish them. They brought us up together. My aunt had more time, she lived with us from the day I was born until I was four years old.

Describing the personality of the parent figure gave respondents the opportunity to compare the various adults that made up their parental universe either in positive terms or in relation to their respective parenting skills.

The notion of "replacement" appeared in several expressions (Table 4.9) relating to experience of both complementary and surrogate parenting.

> On the subject of a maternal aunt: "There were a lot of us at home. Paula wanted to take me because I ate better. She was like a second mother."

Replacement did not exclusively concern orphans but related to a temporary or permanent reassignment of parental functions to these third parties who "played the role" of parents to make up for absence, (during war or following separation or death), lack of availability when the family was large or when the parents' occupations (especially those of the mother) were very demanding,[20] or inadequate care if the parents were "ill", "depressed" or had abandoned their children, either literally or figuratively.[21]

Of course, the composition and functioning of the parental universe also depended on the available resources and each individual's personal availability, a fact which respondents also referred to:

> Thus on the subject of a maternal uncle: "He was a bachelor, we all lived on the same farm. He didn't marry so that he could look after his parents and his sister (my mother) and her three children (us). He devoted himself to us, he was the head of the family and played the role of the missing father." (Quote from a male respondent)

Here the uncle takes on the father's role in a fatherless family because he is a man and his own history is marked by his role, but also because he is available: he lives on the spot, he is not married and has no children. Thus geographic proximity, gender relations, availability in terms of the parent figure's own family and working life, are all important parameters affecting their availability as parental substitutes.

In some cases the terms of comparison are more explicit and the biological parents are compared unfavourably with the complementary or surrogate parent figures:

> On the subject of a childminder: "In terms of affection, she replaced my mother. [She was a] very good person, devoted, had a heart of gold. [I never received] any affection from my mother. I was very sad to return to her because Germaine fell sick. I called her Mummy, I couldn't call my mother Mummy."
>
> Referring to a maternal grandmother: "I lived with her, I was very happy, in the countryside, nice people, she was a mother to me, whereas I was one too many as far as my mother was concerned. My grandmother brought me up."

Lastly, there was the legitimation function, whereby a substitute parent assumed the legal responsibilities of a biological parent in his/her absence. This was mentioned for legally-recognized foster families, as well as for certain figures (usually male) such as uncles, brothers and godfathers. It arose in relation to the respondent's civil status or to the duties of adults as the respondent's official representative in dealings with social services or schools or in precise situations sometimes outside the specific context of childhood (e.g. marriage), and likewise to their duties as the respondent's legal guardian or as the person viewed as his/her protector. When the statement specified that the guardian was "legal" he or she was described in formal, administrative terms. For instance, one respondent said of a paternal uncle who lived locally, "He was not our guardian but he took care of the family and the business like a guardian." However, he specified that, "he didn't live with us so the other brother was more important." This example reveals that the very selective recognition of a parental role from the respondents' viewpoint was based more on practical day-to-day parenting than on the legal role. Guardianship and legitimation were minimized and reduced to an abstract legal function. Conversely, they were valued by respondents when attributed to a person recognized as being a "real" guardian,

[20] In the context, namely from the 1930s to the 1960s, before any form of collective childcare was available.

[21] When the child felt unloved.

even without having any legal status, because those people were present and influential on a daily basis.

Like legal guardians, although the godparents' relationship was formally instituted in law and/or by the parents, they were not necessarily recognized as having a parent function by the child. As a result, this type of relation remained outside the register of practical parenting that prevailed in respondents statements, a fact which explains the limited presence of godparents among the persons mentioned as having played a parental role (Table 4.2 and note 6).

4.4.5 The Special Role of the Grandmother

Grandmothers are dominant parent figures in several respects. They were available, since their own children had grown up, they were often economically inactive, and were very frequently mentioned by respondents, particularly by women (Table 4.10). This calls for a specific examination of their role.

Grandmothers were abundantly described and characterized by the diversity of the functions they held. In the material sphere (using the following terms: *running* [the household], *providing*, *ingredient*, *kitchen*, *preparing*, *care*, *contagious*) as well as in the psychological and intellectual sphere (*share*, *cheerful*, *museum*, *learning about things*, *available*). The grandmother is specifically associated with concocting tasty dishes. She is a cake-making granny but also the mistress of the house who runs the household. The grandmother pays a more important role for the elder children. She is the first figure to be mentioned as a replacement for an absent working mother. Her affective and psychological role is often described as making up for a less affectionate mother. In comparison, information relating to the grandfather, associated first and foremost with the image of the father and the status of the grandmother's husband, is very scant.

Among relatives, the grandmother was most often cited for nurturing functions in early-age experiences, while the childminder was most cited among the non-relatives. The grandmother was also at the top of the list of family figures having an educational role.[22] When respondents described this role they referred to an educational style (*strict*, or on the contrary, *lenient* and *affectionate*), in the precise framework of school work or broader intellectual discovery (*museums*, *reading*, etc.).

Above all, the grandmother was referred to in connection with everyday life. However, the relationship with the grandmother, more than with other parent figures, was viewed as being part of a tradition. Her role often conveys a notion of family transmission. Reference to a female family culture is perceptible, and sometimes set against the relationship between respondents and their own mothers. The grandmother-granddaughter relationship, more than any other, may make up for a difficult relationship between respondents and their mothers, though it may also be in competition (an overbearing grandmother attempting to "squeeze out" the mother).

[22] As were godmothers and godfathers for non-relatives.

4.5 Conclusion

In this article we have presented parent figures from a new angle, based on the viewpoint of the child rather than the adult who occupied or delegated that role. Our analysis is based on the childhood recollections of respondents born between 1930 and 1950. Seen from this new perspective, an unexpected picture of the parental universe emerges:

- One respondent in five mentioned the presence of at least one additional parent figure in his/her childhood. Grandparents, and more specifically the maternal grandmother, were most frequently cited, though the broad range of parent figures referred to – 16 % of whom were not related – is interesting.
- Details of the composition of respondents' parental universes before age 15 reveal that 54 % of respondents grew up in continuous residence with both biological parents; half the respondents who were separated for at least 1 year from both their parents spent a period in boarding school while the other half was entrusted to a third party (usually a grandparent).

An examination of the functions attributed to these "elective parents" highlights the very tangible nature of the care they provided. Strong affective ties with the respondents, and the practical functions of parenting constitute the two criteria for identifying a parent figure, whether or not they belonged to the family circle.

Elective multi-parenting was above all practical. It reflects the parenting role as it was performed and perceived by respondents when they were children. While men described it in general terms, women mentioned personality and the characteristics of the relationship with the individuals concerned.

The grandmother's role stands out. For the cohorts in this study, she was the first person mentioned as making up for the absence of a working mother. She appears as someone who is both attentive and available, as well as the mistress of the house who manages everything in the household. The Second World War period experienced by one segment of the cohorts was characterized by a greater presence of non-related individuals. Over the study period, parent figures began to appear earlier and their influence lasted longer, reflecting the changes due to urbanization and the entry of mothers into the workforce before government policy made life easier for working women.

This practical approach to parenting offers an original perspective that reveals the role and elective aspect of multi-parenting. Indissociable from the feelings of affection that abound in the citations and the explanations of how adult roles were distributed, this elective construction of complementary and, in some cases, substitute parent figures is mirrored in the observation of contemporary family transformations (Fine 2001; Théry 1998).

Appendix

An example of the questionnaire page devoted to collecting information about persons who have played a parental role for the respondent

(see a copy of the complete questionnaire in Chap. 2

Y-a-t-il des PERSONNES ayant joué pour vous un RÔLE PARENTAL ?

Prénom : MARCELINE **Sexe :** (F2) M1 **Lien :** GRAND-MÈRE MATERNELLE

Quelle est la succession des événements familiaux : mise en ménage, mariage, enfants, etc., qui jalonnent sa vie d'adulte ?
(les noter en ordre chronologique)

M E E V *Début de Relation* DC

43

À quelle période son influence a-t-elle été déterminante ? *(enfance, adolescence, jeunesse etc.)*

PENDANT MON ENFANCE JUSQU'À SON DÉCÈS de 5 ans à 7 ans.

HABp **À cette époque, résidait-il (elle) :**

(0.) Avec vous **100.** Dans la même commune ou limitrophe, laquelle : ……

Ailleurs : commune, département (pays) ……

FREp **Quelle était alors la fréquence de vos contacts ?** ……

Pourquoi cette personne a-t-elle été importante ? En quoi a-t-elle joué un rôle parental pour vous ?

Pendant cette période, elle nous a apporté + d'affection que nos parents. Beaucoup d'humour. Elle détendait l'atmosphère.

AP **Pour vous quelle a été son activité principale** *(préciser la qualification, OS, OQ …)* **?**
AGRICULTRICE

(1.) Indépendant(e) **2.** Salarié(e) du secteur public et nationalisé *(préciser)* ……

3. Salarié(e) secteur privé **4.** Autre *(préciser)* ……

Activité de son entreprise : AGRICULTURE
(ex : aviation ; usine ou transport)

HAB **Actuellement (ou avant son décès), cette personne habite-t-elle :** (0.) Avec vous → *Page suivante*

100. Dans la même commune ou limitrophe, laquelle : ……

Ailleurs : commune, département (pays) ……

FRE **Actuellement (ou avant son décès), quelle est (était) la fréquence de vos contacts ?** ……

References

Attias-Donfut, C., Lapierre, N., & Segalen, M. (2002). *Le nouvel esprit de famille*. Paris: O Jacob. 294 p.

Brady, I. (Ed.). (1976). *Transactions in kinship, adoption and fosterage in Oceania* (ASAO monograph 4). Honolulu: Hawaii University Press.

Burguière, A. (1993). De la famille en miettes à la famille recomposée. In M. T. Meulders-Klein & I. Théry (Eds.), *Les recompositions familiales aujourd'hui*. Paris: Nathan (coll. Essais et Recherches).

Chalvon-demersay, S. (1996). Une société élective. Scénarios pour un monde de relations choisies. *Terrain, 27*, 81–100.

Clément, C. (2009). *La mère et ses enfants. Devenir adulte et transmissions intergénérationnelles*. Paris: L'Harmattan, Coll. Populations.

Downs, L. L. (2002). *Childhood in the Promised Land. Working-class movements and the Colonies de Vacances in France, 1880–1960*. Durham/London: Duke University Press.

Downs, L. L. (2005). Milieu social or milieu familial? Theories and practices of childrearing among the popular classes in 20th century France and Britain: The case of evacuation (1939–1945). *Family and Community History, 8*(2), 49–66.

Fine, A. (Ed.). (1998). *Adoptions. Ethnologie des parentés choisies*. Paris: Éditions de la Maison des sciences de l'homme. 309 p.

Fine, A. (2001). Pluriparentalités et systèmes de filiation dans les sociétés occidentales. In L. Gall (Ed.), *Les pluriparentalités dans les sociétés occidentales*. Paris: Puf.

Gollac, S. (2003). Maisonnée et cause commune: une prise en charge familiale. In F. Weber, S. Gojard, & A. Gramain (Eds.), *Charges de famille. Parenté et dépendance dans la France contemporaine*. Paris: La Découverte (coll. Textes à l'appui – Enquêtes de terrain).

Goody, E. (1999). Sharing and transferring components of parenthood: The West African case. In M. Corbier (Ed.), *Adoption and fosterage* (pp. 369–388). Paris: de Boccard.

Lallemand, S. (2002). Familles recomposées : la loi et non l'exception. In J.-F. Dortier (Ed.), *Familles: permanence et métamorphoses*. Auxerre: Éditions Sciences humaines.

Langevin, A. (1989). La mémoire double. *Informations sociales, 4*, 42–46.

Lelièvre, É., & Vivier, G. (2001). Évaluation d'une collecte à la croisée du quantitatif et du qualitatif, l'enquête Biographies et entourage. *Population, 56*(6), 1043–1074.

Lelièvre, É., & Vivier, G. (2006). Les figures parentales dans Biographies et entourage. In *Enfants d'aujourd'hui. Diversité des contextes, pluralité des parcours*, Proceedings of the Aidelf seminar held in Dakar, 10–13 December 2002, Vol. 2, INED, PUF, Paris, pp. 185–194.

Lelièvre, É., Vivier, G., & Clément, C. (2005). Entourage parental: pluriparentalités et confiages des enfants en France entre 1930 et 1970. In K. Vignikin & P. Vimard (Eds.), *Familles au Nord, familles au Sud* (pp. 69–90). Academia-Bruylant/L'Harmattan, Louvain la Neuve, Paris.

Mogoutov, A., & Vichnevskaia, T. (2006). Présentation de la technique d'analyse des données d'enquête sous Réseau-Lu. In M. Loenzien & S.-D. Yana (Eds.), *Les approches qualitatives dans les études de population. Théorie et pratique*. Paris: AUF.

Ouelette, F.-R. (1998). Les usages contemporains de l'adoption. In A. Fine (Ed.), *Adoptions. Ethnologie des parentés choisies* (pp. 153–177). Paris: Éditions de la Maison des sciences de l'homme.

Théry, I. (1998). *Couple, filiation et parenté aujourd'hui: le droit face aux mutations de la famille et de la vie privée* (Rapport à la ministre de l'Emploi et de la Solidarité et au garde des Sceaux, ministre de la Justice). Paris: O. Jacob/La Documentation française. 413 p.

Weber, F. (2003). Pour penser la parenté contemporaine. In D. Debordeaux & P. Strobel (Eds.), *Les solidarités familiales en questions, entraide et transmission*. Paris: LGDJ (Droit et société).

Chapter 5
Memory, Perception of Life, and Family Environment

Valérie Golaz and Éva Lelièvre

5.1 Introduction

Life-event history surveys dealing with the entire life course collate factual data on a wide variety of themes, treated systematically (GRAB 1999). As these surveys are often conducted retrospectively, the influence of memory – given its selective nature – is an important issue (Auriat 1996). Methodological work on the *Triple biographie* survey (Courgeau 1985; Poulain et al. 1991) demonstrated the reliability of retrospective life-event history data collected with appropriate questionnaires and know-how. Errors concerning the exact dates of events do not affect the results as long as the chronological sequence is respected (Courgeau and Lelièvre 1992, pp. 18–26). Retrospective data collection also raises the issue of subjective – possibly idealized – reconstruction: both qualitative and quantitative approaches are susceptible to "smoothing" of life course events. This issue is discussed in detail in the chapter on facts and perceptions in a volume by the Discussion Group on the Event History Approach (*Groupe de réflexion sur l'approche biographique*, GRAB) at INED (GRAB 2009). However, by collating multiple aspects of life histories, quantitative event history data collection reduces the likelihood that respondents will isolate and give preference to particular events over others. Unlike the qualitative recording of life histories, which respects respondents' silence on certain topics or certain periods of their lives – a silence that may speak louder than words (Randall and Koppenhaver 2004) –, quantitative event history data collection seeks to reconstruct a factual sequence of events independently of the subjective perceptions woven into the respondent's discourse (Lelièvre et al. 2009).

This chapter was first published in French in *Mémoire et démographie, regards croisés au Sud et au Nord*, Richard Marcoux and J. Dion (eds.), 2009, Québec, Presses de l'Université Laval, coll. "Cahiers du CIEQ", pp. 155–167.

V. Golaz • É. Lelièvre (✉)
Institut national d'études démographiques (INED), Paris, France
e-mail: eva@ined.fr

C. Bonvalet, É. Lelièvre (eds.), *Family Beyond Household and Kin*,
INED Population Studies 6, DOI 10.1007/978-3-319-24684-0_5

Going beyond the retrospective reconstitution of life-course events, this chapter aims to shed light on the way facts affect perceptions: how a family situation at one point in time affects the way individuals remember these specific moments later in their life. This chapter investigates respondents' subjective assessments of the different periods of their lives and how they tie in with the characteristics of their family environment at the time.

More specifically, the characteristics of individuals' family environment over the course of their lives are matched against respondents' perceptions of their past. The combination of these two retrospective aspects – one factual and one subjective – is an original approach to the issue of selective memory. Do respondents perceive times when they had less family around them as having been more difficult? Do changes in the number of family members around them alter respondents' assessment of the quality of their lives? Does living with both parents have an impact on respondents' perception of their childhoods? How do adults perceive the stages when their children were born, and when they left home? Should the family environment considered for these questions be limited to members of the household or extended to the broader family contact circle? These are the questions addressed in our research. In order to answer them, we first reconstitute the respondents' family contact circles over their lifetimes, i.e. the family members with whom they have lived and the broader group of family contacts. Next, in order to match these data with the subjective assessments of the various stages in their lives identified by the respondents themselves, indicators are devised to describe each period. Last, two different life stages are analysed in this chapter: childhood/adolescence and adulthood.

5.2 Reconstituting Family Contact Circles and Perception of Life over the Course of a Lifetime

Biographies et entourage is a life event history survey conducted in 2001 on a sample of residents of the Paris region born between 1930 and 1950. As well as reconstituting the respondents' lifelong family, residential and occupational trajectories, the survey included a large corpus of data on each respondent's family and friends over his/her lifetime. This "entourage" was defined precisely, prior to data collection, as the people who co-resided with the respondent, his/her direct ascendants and descendants, collateral relatives and spouses, as well as any other individuals described as having played an important role at any time in the respondent's life (Bonvalet and Lelièvre 1995; Lelièvre et al. 1998). The information collected on the respondent's contact circle therefore comprises the household but also extends beyond it. The survey also recorded respondents' perceptions of their life course. In addition to data collected through closed, factual questions, respondents' own interpretations of the sequence of events in their life course, of landmark events and the overall tones of their life histories were noted down (Laborde et al. 2007).

To move from the study of individual trajectories to those of a group of individuals, the principles of observation and analysis applied in life event history surveys

(GRAB 1999) and in surveys of sociability networks (Bonvalet et al. 1993) must be extended and systematized. To make this transition from the individual to the group in a lifelong perspective in the *Biographies et entourage* survey, we decided not only to collect data from a reference person in the group but also to systematically map out a network of key persons over the life course (Lelièvre and Vivier 2001).

5.2.1 Describing the Contact Circle

Describing the contact circle in the survey thus involved identifying a clearly delimited circle of people around the respondent who could be tracked throughout his/her trajectory, including at times when some members did not live with the respondent. This circle therefore consisted of certain *mandatory relatives*, all *co-residents* (related and unrelated) with whom the respondent has lived for at least a year, as well as *significant others* spontaneously cited by the respondent as having played a parental role or having had an important positive or negative influence on his/her life (Inset 1).

Inset 1. Individuals in the Respondent's Contact Circle Identified in the *Biographies et entourage* Survey

Within the family

In direct line:

- ascendants: grandparents, biological parents or adoptive parents, and parents' spouses
- collateral relatives: siblings, half-siblings and foster siblings
- descendants: children and grandchildren

Step relatives:

- life partners (whether married or not, whether co-resident or not)
- partners' parents
- partners' children

Beyond the family

Significant others:

- individuals who have played a parental role for the respondent
- friends, colleagues and other members of the extended family considered by the respondent to have played an important role, whether positive or negative

Systematically through the respondent's life:

- all individuals (whether related or not) with whom the respondent has co-resided for at least a year.

We thus collected information (with varying amounts of detail) about the trajectories of two generations around the respondent (parents and children). We also have information about two additional generations (the respondent's grandparents and grandchildren), as well as about non-relatives whom the respondent considers close. Non-mandatory relatives (uncles, aunts and extended in-laws) only appear in the database if they co-resided with the respondent or if the respondent cited them as having played an important role, parental or otherwise.

Using the recorded information on these trajectories and the type of relationship between the respondent and the individuals close to him/her, we were thus able to reconstitute the respondent's closer family contact circle over the course of his/her life, forming a group that varied in size, ranging from the members of the co-resident family to the broader family circle. This reconstitution was done in the same way for all respondents using data from the questionnaire and did not rely solely on memory, since the questions did not require the respondents to identify their family circle themselves.

5.2.2 Assessing Different Periods of Life

In the *Biographies et entourage* survey, the events that punctuated respondents' lives were recorded, but not their motivations. When the questionnaire had been completed, the respondents were therefore asked to look at the tables where the chronology of family, residential and occupational events was recorded and to divide their lives into periods. They were then invited to "justify" or "explain" each of the periods they identified (Laborde et al. 2007).

Inset 2. Questions Sy1 and Sy2 in ***Biographies et entourage***

Sy1 – Can you divide your life into different periods? Describe each period, by identifying what makes it different from the other periods and what it represents in your life.

Sy2 – Please indicate for each period whether it represented:

- VG very good years
- G good years
- OK problem-free years
- D difficult years
- VD very difficult years

Respondents identified an average of four periods, and one-third of respondents divided their life course into three to five periods (Inset 2). In all, the *Biographies et entourage* survey produced a total of 11,951 life stages.

The distribution of respondents' assessments shows that their trajectories are viewed as positive overall: more than half of all periods were rated "good" or "very good" (Table 5.1). On average, 37 years, i.e. two-thirds of the length of the

Table 5.1 Distribution of assessments given by the respondents to qualify the different periods in their life course

	VG	G	OK	D	VD	Total
Number	2943	3897	1788	2403	920	11,915
Percentage	24.6	32.6	15	20.1	7.7	100
Average length of period assessed (years)	15.9	21.1	9.5	8.7	3.0	58.2

Source: Laborde et al. 2007
Coverage: All respondents who answered the question (N=2799 men and women living in the Paris region aged 50–70)
Interpretation: 24.6 % of periods were rated VG (very good)

trajectories, are rated positively. An age breakdown reveals that good and very good years are not concentrated in a specific time of life. We do not observe, for example, a polarization of positive assessments in the respondents' childhood or youth. The distribution of "good years" across the trajectories reveals the value and validity of these retrospective subjective assessments, which are more complex than a conventional or idealized reconstruction of certain periods of life (such as a golden age of childhood, for example). Slightly over one-quarter of assessments are negative and refer to "difficult" or "very difficult" years (Laborde et al. 2007).

On the whole, the respondents' assessments are very definite: the extreme indicators ("very good"/"very difficult") account for as much as 32 %, i.e. one third of the assessments, while the more neutral indicator ("problem-free"), which is the middle value here, is much less frequent (15 %).

This assessment of past periods of life can be used in the analysis as it stands. By contrast, the respondents' family entourage needs further construction.

5.3 Reconstituting Relations with Close Family over the Life Course

Based on the available information about the respondent's entourage, we are more specifically interested in the close family, i.e. the members of the family closest to the respondent genealogically, as well as individuals who have played a parental role (Lelièvre and Vivier 2006; Lelièvre et al. 2008). In all, therefore, close family comprises: parents and other individuals who have played a parental role, siblings, spouses and children. Although not all close family members necessarily have a close relationship with the respondent, we assume that they have all had an influence on the respondent's trajectory.

We consider two conceptions of the close family. The first is the most restricted conception, consisting of close family members who are co-residing with the respondent. The *co-resident close family* can be considered as the smallest group that influences the respondent. We can map its characteristics accurately over the respondent's life by using the life event history table from the questionnaire, one section of which is devoted to all the individuals (related and unrelated) who have lived with the respondent for at least a year.

However, in order to include non-co-resident members of the close family in our study, we also defined the close family network, which consists of all family members who are in frequent contact with the respondent each year of his/her past life. The *close family network* thus includes the co-resident close family but extends beyond that inner circle to family members who remain in contact and whose influence persists throughout the respondent's trajectory. Alongside the periods of co-residence, various sections of the database are used to reconstitute this family network:

- information on each of these individuals, such as the person's birth and death, or the frequency of contact with the respondent at the time of the survey, and the period of influence of individuals cited as having played a parental role;
- the geographical proximity of the respondent's and his/her parents' places of residence, from the respondent's birth until the time of the survey.

The available data are not sufficient to estimate the presence or absence of contact between the respondent and each of these individuals at all times in his/her past life. Ahead of the analysis, we therefore have to address the problem of missing information. Assumptions are made, based on the amount of information we have about the individual in question and his/her relationship to the respondent.

The close family network was thus reconstituted on the basis of three assumptions:

- A1. Between periods of co-residence with the respondent, they remain in contact;
- A2. Individuals enter the close family network at the following times: by birth in the case of direct descendants and siblings; 1 year before the start of the conjugal relationship in the case of life partners, assuming that meeting and dating precede the start of the conjugal relationship; or in the year mentioned by the respondent for other parental figures;
- A3. Individuals leave the close family network in most cases through death or the breakdown of relationships, i.e. when frequency of contact falls to below four times per year. If a relationship has ended by the time of the survey, we assume that this coincides with the end of co-residence for children, siblings, adopted parents and parents' spouses, whereas for biological parents we use the date when they no longer reside in the same or a neighbouring municipality. For spouses, we estimate that breakdown occurs in the year of divorce, or in the year of separation if the spouses do not divorce. For other parental figures, the end of the period of influence cited by the respondent is accepted.

We were thus able to construct two databases, which, for each year of the respondent's life, indicate the size and structure of a group of related people centred around the respondent, i.e. close family in its restricted composition (the co-resident close family) and its broad composition (the close family network).

The average size of the co-resident close family of respondents born between 1930 and 1950 and residing in the Paris region varies with the respondent's age (Fig. 5.1). It is largest at around age 10, when it consists of almost four people on average (slightly fewer than two parents/slightly fewer than two siblings). After shrinking around age 25, the co-resident close family grows again up to age 35. The departure of siblings is counterbalanced by the arrival of a spouse and children. Children leave in turn when the respondent is aged between 40 and 65. At age 70, respondents live on average with one other person from their close family.

The close family network of residents of the Paris region born between 1930 and 1950 increased from an average of four people during childhood to more than five people between 30 and 50, then fell gradually to below four people around age 70 (Fig. 5.2). The respondents' siblings and children make up the bulk of the close family network over the entire life course. From ages 0 to 25, the network consists mainly of the biological parents and siblings, and from 30 onwards, children account for the largest relative share (Fig. 5.2). The average network size varies relatively little over the course of a lifetime, and at age 70, respondents are still in frequent contact with an average of four close family members.

The numbers of ascendants and collateral relatives are very similar for men and women at every stage of life. However, there are noticeable gender differences when it comes to the number of spouses and children in the close family. On average, women form unions younger than men, and the percentage of women who no longer live with a spouse steadily increases from age 35 onwards (Fig. 5.3). Similarly, the percentage of women who are in regular contact with a spouse or former spouse also diminishes (Fig. 5.4). By contrast, the same percentage of men live with a spouse at age 60 as at age 40. Children are born earlier in women's trajectories than in men's (Fig. 5.3), and it is not until age 50 that fathers and mothers have the same average number of children in their entourage (Fig. 5.4).

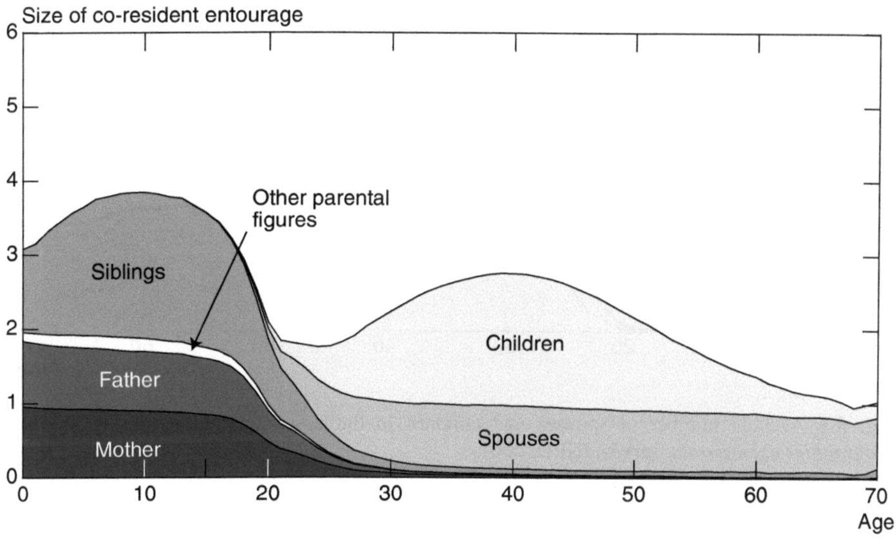

Fig. 5.1 Average size of co-resident close family (*Source*: *Biographies et entourage* survey, INED, 2001)

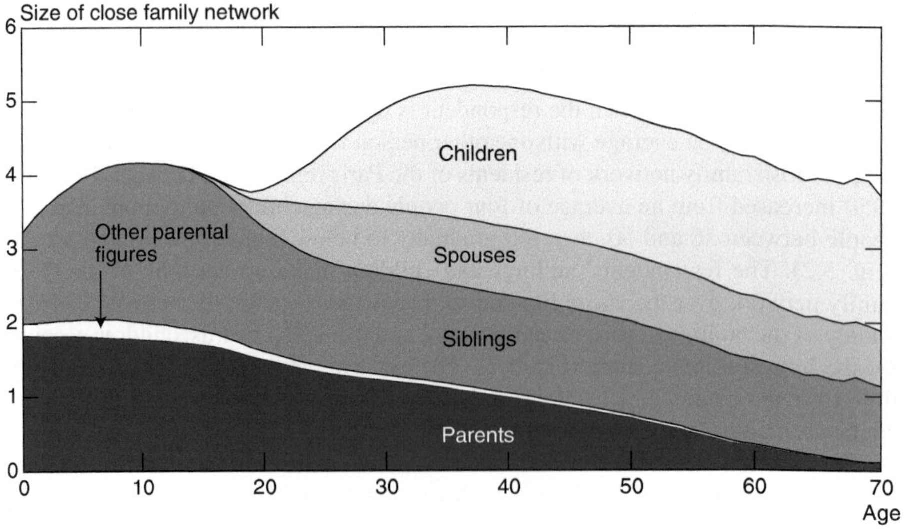

Fig. 5.2 Average size of close family network (*Source*: *Biographies et entourage* survey, INED, 2001)

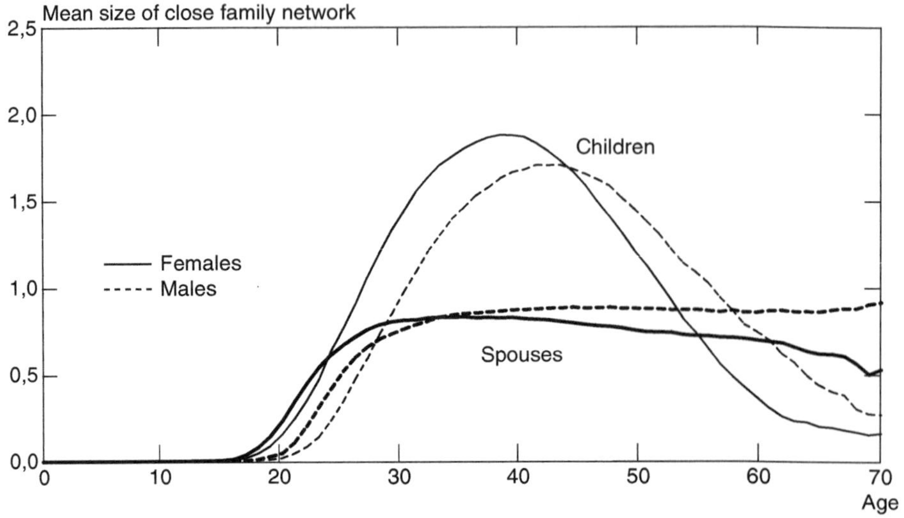

Fig. 5.3 Average number of spouses and children in the co-resident close family (*Source*: *Biographies et entourage* survey, INED, 2001)

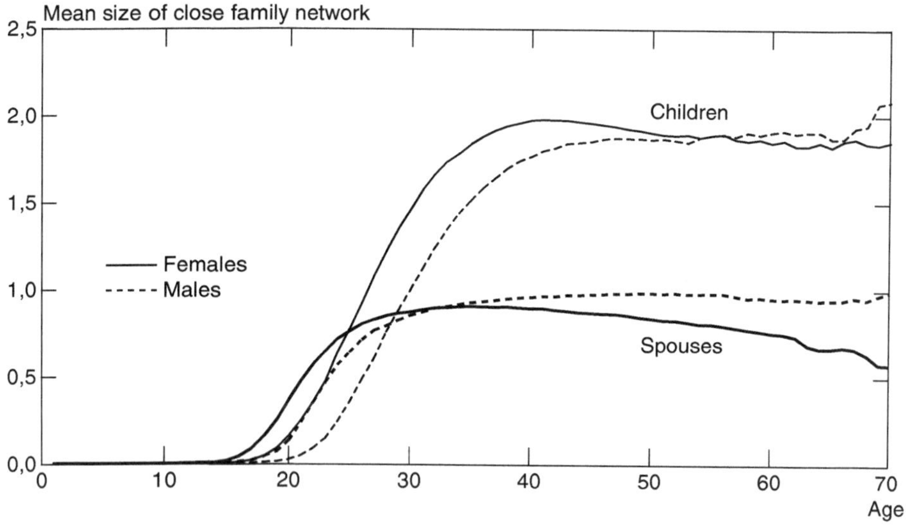

Fig. 5.4 Average number of spouses and children in the close family network (*Source*: *Biographies et entourage* survey, INED, 2001)

5.4 Modelling the Impact of Family on Assessment of the Period of Life

In practical terms, in order to match the composition of the respondent's family entourage over his/her lifetime – defined as his/her co-resident close family or close family network – against the respondent's assessments of the periods he/she has identified, the analysis must focus on these periods. Thus, after reconstituting the respondent's close family for each year of his/her life, we next developed indicators to summarize the characteristics of the close family and changes to it in each of the life periods assessed. As the tone of a period is rated by respondents *ex-post*, and in general terms for the entire period delimited by the survey, it makes no sense to attribute this rating to each year of the period. We are not interested here in an event history approach or in the actual length of the period. Rather, our aim is to consider these periods as defined by the respondents at a specific time in their trajectory (i.e. at the time of the survey) and to match the respondent's assessment of each one against the characteristics of his/her entourage at the time, reconstituted from the factual data gathered in the survey. The statistical unit investigated here is thus the subjective period. The 2830 respondents to the *Biographies et entourage* survey defined a total of 11,951 periods. For each period, we calculated several indicators to describe, in as much detail as possible, the size and structure of the respondent's close family.

5.4.1 Indicators of the Size of the Close Family during a Given Period

- Average size of the close family during the period
- Standard deviation of the size of the close family during the period
- Change in the size of the close family during the period:

  increasing monotone
  decreasing monotone
  non-monotone
  constant

5.4.2 Indicators of the Structure of the Close Family during a Given Period

- No spouse in the close family during the period
- A spouse leaves the close family during the period
- No children in the close family during the period
- A child leaves the close family during the period
- Presence of siblings during the period, and presence of more than two siblings
- No parents for at least 1 year of the period, and both parents for the whole period
- Presence of other individuals who played a parental role

Moreover, because the size and composition of the entourage is heavily dependent on both the life period and the respondent's sex, we decided to conduct our analysis separately for periods that were relatively homogeneous, studying men and women independently. We thus worked in detail on the episodes occurring within two broad life stages:

- *Childhood and adolescence*: all episodes ending before the respondent's 21st birthday (N = 2840 episodes)
- *Adulthood*: all episodes beginning after the respondent's 21st birthday (N = 6277 episodes)[1]

The next two sections present the results of logistic regressions explaining the influence of the characteristics of the respondents' close family on their assessment of the periods of childhood/adolescence and adulthood (Tables 5.2 and 5.3). In the models, the statistical unit is the period. The dependent variable is the assessment of the period as "difficult" or "very difficult". Each time, the two extreme definitions

[1] The episodes that began in childhood and ended in adulthood were not taken into account, which leads to a slight over-representation of difficult periods (the shortest) compared with positively assessed periods (the longest). However, we assume here that this has a negligible impact on the models used.

Table 5.2 Direction of link between difficult periods and variables of the models for childhood and adolescence[a]

	Model 1	Model 2
Assessment	Co-resident close family	Close family network
Negative	Neither parent present (M & W)	Neither parent present (M & W)
	Only one parent present (M & W)	Only one parent present (M & W)
	Other parental figure(s) present (M)	Other parental figure(s) present (M)
Positive	1936–1950 cohorts (M)	1936–1950 cohorts (M)
	Length of period (M & W)	Length of period (M & W)
	Born in France (M)	Born in France (M)

(M) Men (W) Women
[a]The full table is given in the appendix (Table A.1)

Table 5.3 Direction of link between difficult periods and variables of the models for adulthood[a]

	Model 1	Model 2
Assessment	Co-resident close family	Close family network
Negative	*Decreasing size of close family (W)*[b]	*Strong variance in size of close family (M)*
	No child at home (W)	*Departure of a child (W)*
	Departure of a spouse (M & W)	Departure of a spouse (M & W)
Positive	Length of period (M & W)	Length of period (M & W)
	Small close family (M)	Increasing size of close family (M & W)
	Increasing size of close family (M & W)	Born in provincial France (M).
	Born in provincial France (M)	*Non-monotone size of close family (W)*
	Departure of a child (W)	*Presence of a spouse (W)*
	Presence of a spouse (M & W)	

[a]The full table is given in the appendix (Table A.2)
[b](M) Men (W) Women. The variables in italics highlight the differences between the two models

of close family are tested: the co-resident close family and the close family network. In each of the models presented here, control variables related to the respondent (year and place of birth) and to the characteristics of the period (its length) were introduced. In every case, the length of the period and the respondent's assessment are correlated, with the shortest periods rated as more difficult overall than the longest.

5.5 The Presence of Parental Figures in Periods Assessed as Difficult

In childhood and adolescence (Table 5.2), the respondent's birth cohort is only significant for boys. Boys born between 1936 and 1950 experienced happier episodes overall than boys born between 1930 and 1935. This is probably due to the impact of the Second World War and post-war reconstruction. The 1941–1945 cohorts make the most positive assessment.

Before age 21, the size of the close family is conditioned by the presence of parents and other parental figures. The presence of siblings and the average size of the close family have little influence. Women's assessments of their childhood and adolescence are influenced only by the presence of parents in the household or in the contact circle (the episodes spent with both parents are significantly happier). The presence of other parental figures does not play a significant role for women. The presence of parents in the household or in the contact circle also has an influence on men's assessments, but the presence of parental figures is also significant. Periods in childhood that men rated as difficult are linked to being born abroad and to the presence of parental figures, who may have helped overcome the difficulties experienced.

The main findings of this analysis are the importance of the presence of both parents in the contact circle and in the household, as well as the significance for boys of the presence of other parental figures during periods rated as more difficult than others. We note that the two models are very similar: the results are the same for the co-resident close family and the close family network when we study the links between the close family and the subjective assessment of childhood.

5.6 Assessments of Adulthood Are Strongly Linked to Conjugal Life and Motherhood for Women – And for Women Only

In adulthood (Table 5.3), the cohort effect is not significant. For men, the periods rated as significantly happier than others are those when the co-resident close family includes a spouse but remains small (maximum one spouse and one child). The increasing size of the close family network is also a positive factor, but with no size limit. For men, the close family network may grow if they start a new union and new children are born, changes that correspond to good years, even if separations are reflected in difficult periods.

Women feel positively about periods when the size of the co-resident close family or the family network increases, with no perceptible size limit. However, when we look at the structure of the close family, women rate the periods when a spouse is present as less difficult. Conversely, both women and men assess periods during which a spouse leaves as difficult. Periods when there is at least one child in the household are perceived less positively than others. Combined with the previous results about the speed of change in the size of the close family over the period, this factor shows simply that after the stage of family formation, which is assessed positively overall, come the trials of family life, complicated by difficulties such as poor housing or parental unemployment. Moreover, periods during which a child leaves the household are experienced as significantly better than others (Model 1). Periods are perceived as less difficult when children leave gradually than when a spouse and children leave simultaneously. Moreover, when a child leaves the family network (Model 2), i.e. when a child completely breaks off contact with his/her mother or dies, the period is significantly more difficult. Overall, major changes in the size of the close family network are correlated with difficult periods.

For women, the episodes after age 21 are strongly influenced by conjugal life and children. The periods when children leave the parents' home are assessed positively, whereas the periods when children are present often correspond to more difficult times.

Using two original characteristics drawn from an exceptional source, we have explored one of the factors that influences our memory of different periods in our lives, namely our family environment at the time. The *Biographies et entourage* survey asked respondents about the trajectories of a number of mandatory relatives. These factual data enabled us to reconstitute the co-resident family and, beyond that, the family network, limited here to parents, other individuals who have played a parental role, siblings and children, over the respondents' lifetimes. The composition of the respondent's family environment over the life course was thus not directly identified by him/her at the time of the survey but was reconstituted by collating precisely defined factual information. This mode of construction, while making no claims to universal accuracy, does ensure maximum comparability between respondents.

By contrast, the respondents' assessments of the periods in his/her past life from the *Biographies et entourage* survey are perceptions produced at the time of the survey. They are thus subjective and unique (Lelièvre et al. 2009).

What do we learn from this comparison of facts with the perceptions of those facts? The analysis above suggests several ideas for further research that would be worth pursuing.

Firstly, the analysis shows that perceptions of the past are strongly conditioned by the respondent's sex. In the family sphere, men's perceptions seem more dependent on their relationships with their parents and their spouses, whereas women's perceptions are less sensitive to parents and strongly influenced by children. Aside from the interpretation of that finding, men and women do not remember their past in the same way. For example, the Second World War does not show up statistically in women's assessments of their childhood, whereas it is perceptible in men's.

The analysis also shows that not only do the household members have a significant influence on respondents' assessments, but that close family members in contact with the respondent are also important in adulthood.

Relying by definition on memory, retrospective surveys depend upon respondents' recall of past events. These results show the value of comparing direct perception with factual reconstitution. First, factors outside the strict framework of individual states and events from birth to the time of the survey recorded in a life event history table, such as the trajectories of family members, also appear to be important. Second, when perceptions are studied, the factors that influence those perceptions need to be tested before seeking to interpret their meaning. Subjective assessments are dependent on a number of factors, which we are only beginning to identify here.

5.7 Appendices

Table A.1 Relative probability of experiencing a difficult period in childhood or adolescence

	Co-resident close family				Close family network			
Variables	Men		Women		Men		Women	
Respondent's year of birth								
1930–1935	*Ref.*		ns	ns	*Ref.*		ns	ns
1936–1940	−0.42	*	ns	ns	−0.39	*	ns	ns
1941–1945	−0.67	***	ns	ns	−0.62	**	ns	ns
1946–1950	−0.48	**	ns	ns	−0.48	**	ns	ns
Place of birth								
Paris region	−0.47	*	ns	ns	−0.42	*	ns	ns
Provincial France	−0.33	*	ns	ns	−0.28	ns	ns	ns
Abroad or French overseas territory	Ref.		ns	ns	*Ref.*		ns	ns
Length of period								
Short	0.56	**	0.61	***	0.64	***	0.80	***
Medium	*Ref.*		*Ref.*		*Ref.*		*Ref.*	
Long	−0.41	**	−0.53	***	−0.26	ns	−6.23	ns
Number of parents present								
No parent for at least a year	0.87	***	0.39	**	0.48	*	0.35	***
At least one parent, but not both parents for the whole period	0.65	**	0.37	*	0.51	**	0.43	**
Both parents for the whole period	*Ref.*		*Ref.*		*Ref.*		*Ref.*	
Other parental figures								
No other parental figure	−0.40	*	ns	ns	−0.37	*	ns	ns
At least one other parental figure	*Ref.*		ns	ns	*Ref.*		ns	ns

*** significant at 0.1 %; ** at 1 %; * at 5 %; *ns* not significant

Table A.2 Relative probability of experiencing a difficult period in adulthood

Variables	Co-resident close family				Close family network			
	Men		Women		Men		Women	
Place of birth								
Paris region	−0.23	ns	ns	ns	−0.25	ns	ns	ns
Provincial France	−0.40	***	ns	ns	−0.46	***	ns	ns
Abroad or French overseas territory	*Ref.*		ns	ns	*Ref.*		ns	ns
Length of period								
Short	0.50	***	0.60	***	0.42	***	0.50	***
Medium	*Ref.*		*Ref.*		*Ref.*		*Ref.*	
Long	−1.16	***	−1.00	***	−1.03	***	−0.82	***
Speed of change in size of close family during the period								
Increasing monotone	−0.31	**	−0.21	ns	−0.72	***	−0.27	*
Decreasing monotone	−0.14	ns	0.09	ns	−0.37	ns	0.08	ns
Non-monotone	−0.58	***	−0.30	*	−0.88	***	−0.56	***
Constant	*Ref.*		*Ref.*		*Ref.*		*Ref.*	
Variance in size of close family								
High	ns	ns	ns	ns	0.40	*	ns	ns
Average	ns	ns	ns	ns	*Ref.*		ns	ns
Average size of close family								
Small	−0.35	**	ns	ns	ns	ns	ns	ns
Medium	−0.29	*	ns	ns	ns	ns	ns	ns
Large	*Ref.*		ns	ns	ns	ns	ns	ns
Presence of a spouse								
No spouse present during the period	*Ref.*		*Ref.*		ns	ns	*Ref.*	
At least one spouse for at least 1 year	−0.56	***	−0.70	***	ns	ns	−0.53	***
Departure of a spouse								
Spouse does not leave the close family during the period	*Ref.*		*Ref.*		*Ref.*		*Ref.*	
At least one spouse leaves the close family during the period	0.82	***	0.78	***	0.66	***	0.77	***
Presence of children								
No child present during the period	ns	ns	*Ref.*		ns	ns	ns	ns
At least one child present for at least 1 year	ns	ns	0.49	***	ns	ns	ns	ns
Departure of children								
No child leaves the close family during the period	ns	ns	ns	ns	ns	ns	*Ref.*	
At least one child leaves the close family during the period	ns	ns	ns	ns	ns	ns	0.60	**

*** significant at 0.1 %; ** at 1 %; * at 5 %; *ns* non significant

References

Auriat, N. (1996). *Les défaillances de la mémoire humaine*. Paris: INED, coll. Les Cahiers, 136.
Bonvalet, C., & Lelièvre, E. (1995). Du concept de ménage à celui d'entourage: une redéfinition de l'espace familial. *Sociologie et sociétés*, numéro spécial, Une nouvelle morphologie sociale, *27*(2), 177–190.
Bonvalet, C., Maison, D., Le Bras, H., & Charles, L. (1993). Proches et parents. *Population, 48*(1), 83–110.
Courgeau, D. (1985). Interaction between spatial mobility, family and career life-cycle: A French survey. *European Sociological Review, 1*(2), 39–162.
Courgeau, D., & Lelievre, E. (1992). *Event history analysis in demography* (226 p.). Oxford: Clarendon Press/Oxford University Press.
GRAB (Groupe de réflexion sur l'approche biographique). (1999). *Biographies d'enquêtes. Bilan de 14 collectes biographiques*. Paris: INED, coll. Méthodes et savoirs, 3.
GRAB (Groupe de réflexion sur l'approche biographique). (2009). *Fuzzy states: Observing, modelling and interpreting complex trajectories in life histories*, Paris: INED, Méthodes et Savoirs 6 (176 p.).
Laborde, C., Lelièvre, E., & Vivier, G. (2007). Trajectories and landmark events: How people narrate their lives. analysis of life course facts and perceptions. *Population, English Edition, 2*(62), 487–506.
Lelièvre, E., & Vivier, G. (2001). Évaluation d'une collecte à la croisée du quantitatif et du qualitatif, l'enquête Biographies et entourage. *Population, An English Selection, 56*(6), 1043–1074.
Lelièvre, E., & Vivier, G. (2006). "Les figures parentales dans *Biographies et entourage*", actes du colloque de l'Aidelf Dakar 2002, *Enfants d'aujourd'hui, diversité des contextes, pluralité des parcours* (pp. 185–194). Paris: INED.
Lelièvre E., Bonvalet C., & Bry X. (1998). Event history analysis of groups. The findings of an on-going research project. An English selection: *New methodological approaches in the social sciences*, *Population*, 10(1), 11–37.
Lelièvre, E., Vivier, G., & Tichit, C. (2008). Between socially-instituted parental relationships and elective ones: A retrospective analysis of parent figures in France from 1930 to 1965. *Population, English Edition, 2*(63), 209–238.
Lelièvre, E., Roubaud, F., Tichit, C., & Vivier, G. (2009). Factual data and perceptions: Fuzziness in observation and analysis. In *Fuzzy states: Observing, modelling and interpreting complex trajectories in life histories* (pp. 25–54), in GRAB, Paris: INED, Méthodes et Savoirs 6.
Poulain, M., Riandey, B., & Firdion, J. M. (1991). Enquête biographique et registre belge de population: confrontation des données. *Population, 46*(1), 65–88.
Randall, S., & Koppenhaver, T. (2004). Qualitative data in demography. The sound of silence and other problems. *Demographic Research*, MPIDR, 11, article 3, pp. 58–93.

Chapter 6
Family Relationships of Older People

Catherine Bonvalet and Éva Lelièvre

Longer life expectancy is producing a deep shift in the family network, which is now dominated by intergenerational relationships. More and more children now know their grandparents,[1] or even great-grandparents, and a growing percentage of retirees still have living parents. In the 1970s, questions about the continuity of family relationships in industrial societies mainly concerned relationships between parents and their young adult children. Most studies sought to disprove Parsons' theory, by showing that the nuclear family was not isolated from the kinship network and that exchanges and favours continued after children left home. Louis Roussel (1976) and Catherine Gokalp (1978) highlighted the surprising geographical proximity of parents and their adult children, confirming Young and Willmott's pioneering work (1957). In the 1990s, questions arose about the impact of socio-demographic change on family relationships, in a context of economic crisis and challenges to the welfare state. Researchers wondered whether the rise of individualism coincided with weaker mutual support within families. Studies on the extended family increased, and major surveys were conducted in France by INED,[2] INSEE[3] and CNAV.[4] These highlighted the existence of numerous inter-generational relationships, even if the relationships between adult children and their parents are extremely diverse, and in some cases

This article was originally published in *Retraite et sociétés* in "Les Nouvelles données démographiques", 2005, 45, pp. 44–69.

[1] In 1982 H. Le Bras showed that a 20-year-old had two grandparents on average, compared with only 0.14 in the eighteenth century (Le Bras and Roussel 1982).

[2] *Proches et parents* survey (Close circle and parents), see Bonvalet et al. 1993.

[3] *Échanges au sein de la parentèle et des ménages complexes* survey (Exchanges within the kinship and complex households), see Crenner 1998.

[4] *Trois générations* survey (Three generations), see Attias-Donfut 1995.

C. Bonvalet (✉) • É. Lelièvre (✉)
Institut national d'études démographiques (INED), Paris, France
e-mail: bonvalet@ined.fr; eva@ined.fr

C. Bonvalet, É. Lelièvre (eds.), *Family Beyond Household and Kin*,
INED Population Studies 6, DOI 10.1007/978-3-319-24684-0_6

ambivalent. Some adults have distanced themselves from their parents, whereas others maintain very close relationships with their families of origin. At the turn of the twenty-first century, research questions concerned not only the relationships between parents and their married children, but also the role of grandparents in society (Attias-Donfut and Segalen 1998) and the family environment of older people (Delbès and Gaymu 2003), particularly dependent older people (Désesquelles and Brouard 2003).

Those previous studies showed that relationships maintained by older persons with their close circle depend on the joint histories of the family members (Gotman 2007). The study of family relationships must therefore extend well beyond the role of the family as simply a provider of services and social capital.

Some researchers have therefore developed other concepts, such as the entourage, to describe the sociability group, which is the network within which individuals interact over the course of their lives and at the onset of old age. The concept of "*entourage*" is an attempt to broaden the respondents' reference group beyond the network of parents, siblings, children (whether co-resident or not), partners and parents-in-law, to include all the individuals with whom they have co-resided at any time in their life and any significant others, whether related or not, who have played a key role in their lives (Bonvalet and Lelièvre 1995; Lelièvre et al. 1998).

Box 6.1. Testimonies
***Proches et parents* survey**

Christine, from a middle-class family of five children and herself a mother of five, describes her childhood holidays and how she wanted to recreated the same family atmosphere:

> My father and mother bought a family home for us five children, where we spent all our holidays; it was traditional in France to do that. No-one thought of going anywhere else. We spent all of our holidays with… let me see, 14 or 17, well, with all our cousins… I bought a house, which we are currently doing up and my children come there. If you like, we have recreated what my parents did in S., on the other side of the valley in V. So things go on in the same way.

***Biographies et entourage* survey**

A respondent remembers the atmosphere in the construction-site hut on the outskirts of Paris where she lived from 1955 to 1959 with her husband, an electrician on building sites. Despite their uncomfortable lodgings, her grandmother from Brittany came to spend every winter with them:

> She liked living in the hut. She was content. She was happy… She looked after the children. At night we set up a camp bed for her… We unfolded it at night… My grandmother was happy. And so were we.

Later in the interview, the respondent describes the social-housing apartment where she has been living for the past 35 years:

> And our room is Mum's room. We call it Mum's room.

(continued)

Box 6.1 (continued)

Her mother comes to spend every winter there. When she is no longer able to live alone in Brittany, she will come to live with her daughter, "because it will be up to me to take in Mum the way Mum took in Nana. Things come round like that." For the past 8 years, the respondent has also been minding her granddaughter on weekdays.

> And when we go to Brittany to spend the holidays with my other daughter, we take our granddaughter. I take little Julie everywhere with me.

Thus the concept of "entourage" introduced by the *Biographies et entourage* survey provides a means to describe the exchanges between generations, the spatialization of the network and its transformation over time, since the vast majority of respondents have experienced the roles of child and grandchild, parent then grandparent. In this chapter, we deal first with the respondents' relationships with their parents, and with their ascendants more broadly (parents and parents-in-law). Restricting the sample to respondents aged over 60, we also consider their relationships with their children.

This enables us to map out a complete picture, with respondents aged 50–70 in 2000 initially considered in terms of their relationships with their parents, whose life expectancy has increased considerably but who are facing health problems and a loss of autonomy in advanced age; then for the older respondents (those aged 60–70), we examine the sociability they maintain with their children.

6.1 The Family Entourage of Residents of Greater Paris Aged 50–70

6.1.1 Relationships between the Respondents and Their Ascendants

The "family entourage" as documented in this survey of residents of the Paris region observed at the time of the survey can only be understood in relation to the family histories of the different generations that make up the kinship group. The family passes on values cultural capital and social practices, so the dynamics of an older person's network are not independent of the family group in which he/she grew up (the place of grandparents, the number of aunts and uncles, cousins and siblings). In all social classes, we observe this phenomenon of reproduction of the grandparenting style (see Box 6.1. Testimonies).

Before analysing the network at the time of the survey, it is therefore important to examine the affective environment in which these generations grew up. The transmission of social practices and of know-know depends on the type of family in which the respondents lived, and is often passed on by the women. Middle-class, working class and rural families transmit knowledge that differs not only in terms of their occupational skills and assets (*bourgeoisie*) but also in terms of the organization of labour (rural). The roots of some respondents born between 1930 and 1950 go back to the nineteenth century, since their parents were born between 1846 and 1935. They grew up at a time when the image of old age was changing. In France, under the impetus of the government's Laroque Commission (1960–1961), two new images of the "third age" were introduced: integrated old age and autonomous old age. While this change concerned the respondents' parents, some of their grandparents had been dependants and had died before the emergence of this new model (Guillemard 1991).

It is worth remembering that the younger respondents entered adulthood at a time when society was questioning the institution of the family, and young adults were distancing themselves from their parents and grandparents, as attested by publications such as *The Death of the Family* (Cooper 1970) and *Finie la famille?* (Collectif 1975). This makes it all the more interesting to compare the environment of the respondents' youth with the environment they are experiencing now.

The data collected in the *Biographies et entourage* survey about the respondents' parents (date and place of birth, place of residence, year of death if deceased, activities and frequency of contact) and grandparents (living in the household or nearby) are useful for reconstructing the respondents' family environment in their childhood. More conventionally, the data from the survey on places of residence and frequency of contact with parents-in-law enables us to capture the respondents' family environment at the time of the data collection. The survey also provides detailed information about the relationships that the respondents maintain with their children and grandchildren. We are therefore able to compare the family entourage of these cohorts in childhood and adolescence (before age 14) with their entourage at the time of the survey.

The parental environment of these cohorts – one of the components of this entourage – is highly varied (Lelièvre and Vivier 2001. Only 54 % of respondents lived continuously with their biological parents from ages 0 to 14,[5] and a fair number (9 %) lived with their parents and another influential figure in childhood.

A full 21 % of the respondents cited at least one person who played a parental role for them. These parental figures were mostly women (68 %) and the vast majority (87 %) were related to the respondent. The relationships between these people and the respondents are highly varied, reflecting three different generations: 54 % belong to the respondents' grandparents' or even great-grandparents' generation, 25 % belong to the respondents' parents' generation (uncles, aunts and partners) and 8 % belong to the respondents' own generation (siblings and cousins). Consequently, few of these parental figures were still alive at the time of the survey and are not included in the following analysis.

[5] Which does not mean that these respondents all grew up in a nuclear family; other people (grandparents, uncles, aunts, etc.) may have co-resided in the household.

Owing to the respondents' age, many of their parents were already deceased by the time of the survey. According to figures from the *Family Survey* conducted alongside the 1999 French census, a majority of the French population aged over 55 had lost both parents, and almost three-quarters[6] of the population aged 50–54 had lost their fathers (see Table 6.1; see also Monnier and Pennec 2003).

At the time of the survey, more than half (53.8 %) of the residents of the Paris region aged 50–70 had lost both parents. Almost one-third (32.5 %) still had one living parent, usually the mother (in 80 % of cases). Only 14 % of all respondents had both parents living. But the percentage varies considerably between cohorts, ranging from 4 % in the 1930–1940 birth cohorts to 20 % in the 1940–1950 cohorts (see Fig. 6.1).

The average age of the sample of 1695 living parents was 82 years, with the youngest aged 65 and the oldest 106.

Table 6.1 People aged 50–70 in 1999 whose parents were deceased (%)

Age	Father deceased	Mother deceased	Both parents deceased	Total
50–54	36.9	7.4	36.3	80.6
55–59	29.0	5.6	57.4	91.9
60–64	20.3	3.0	74.2	97.6
65–69	12.0	1.5	85.6	99.1

Source: *Étude de l'histoire familiale*, INSEE, 1999

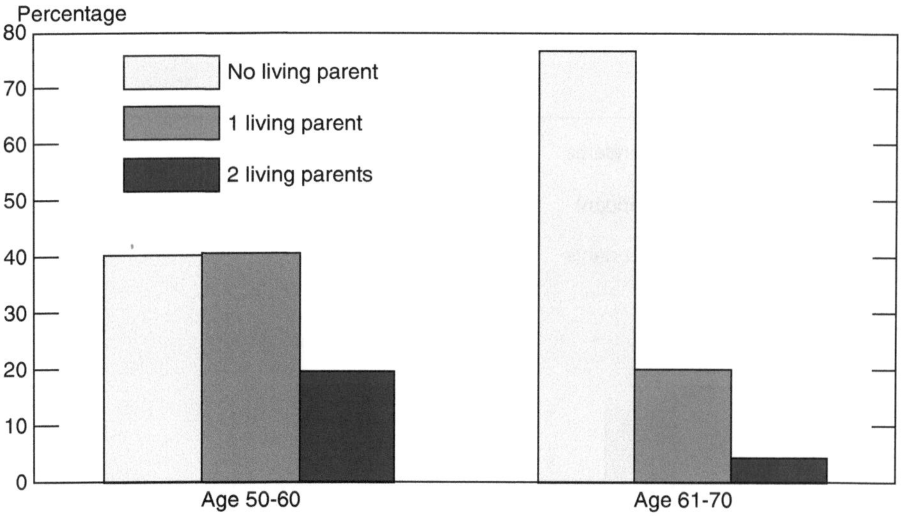

Fig. 6.1 Proportion by age of respondents with living parents (*Source*: *Biographies et entourage* survey, INED, 2001)

[6] Some 36.9 % had lost their father and 36.3 % had lost both parents, making a total of 73.2 %.

6.1.2 Distribution of Ascendants of Respondents Living with a Partner

At the time of the survey, seven out of ten respondents aged 50–70 and living in a couple have at least one living ascendant (parent or parent-in-law) out of the four possible in their family network. When at least one of the partners is under 60 years old, eight out of ten respondents have at least one living ascendant in their network, half have at least two living ascendants and one-fifth at least three.

Among the oldest couples (both partners aged over 60), a majority (55 %) have no ascendants in their family network, 28 % have one living ascendant, and 16 % have two or more (see Fig. 6.2). The gradual disappearance of parents from their family environment is counterbalanced by the appearance of young generations who have left the family home. Indeed, over time, the respondents' parents are replaced by their adult children's independent households, as the respondents themselves become the "elders" of the family.

6.1.3 People Aged over 60 and Their Children

Some 20 % of respondents aged over 60 are still living with at least one of their children, and more than four out of five respondents from the oldest cohorts have at least one child living outside the household. Some have one or two living parents as well as non-co-resident children in their entourage (see Table 6.2). Of the 17 % of

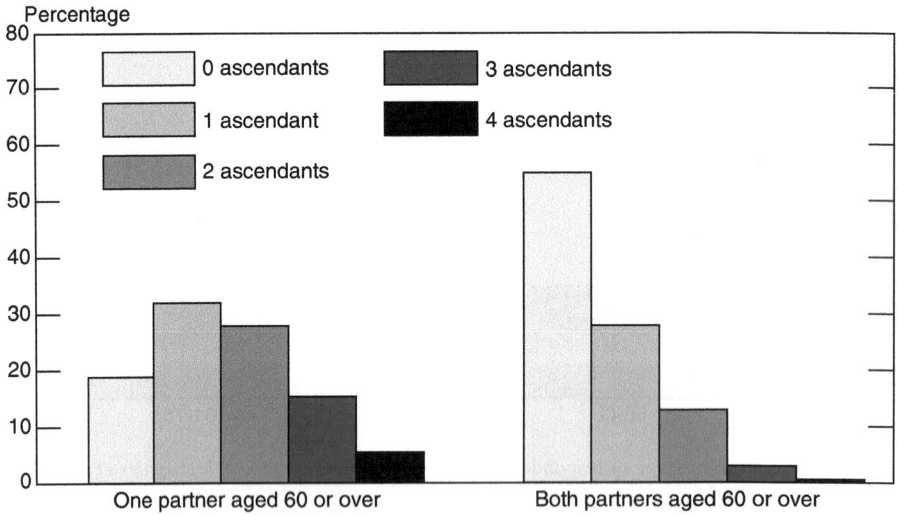

Fig. 6.2 Percentage of living ascendants by partners' ages (*Source*: *Biographies et entourage* survey, INED, 2001)

Table 6.2 Distribution of number of non co-resident children among respondents aged 60+

Non co-resident children	%
None	17
1 child	23
2 children	33
3 children	15
4+ children	12

Source: *Biographies et entourage survey*, INED, 2001
Scope: Residents of Paris region born between 1930 and 1950

respondents aged over 60 with no children living outside the household, the majority (72 %) are childless. The specific position of this generation is clearly apparent: this is the sandwich generation (Attias-Donfut 1995), which has to cope simultaneously with ageing parents who are becoming increasingly dependent, and children who are finding it increasingly difficult to achieve autonomy.

6.2 Residential Proximity of Family Members at the Time of the Survey

The geographical location of the kinship network depends on the family and occupational trajectories of each member of the group. The *Proches et parents* survey showed that a family that lives closed together is more the result of the experiences of several generations and lineages than of demographic and social determinism (Bonvalet 2003). Indeed, as Anne Gotman writes (2007): "the residential space is not independent of the family's history; neither is it confined simply to the primary home; and the residential practices of households can only be understood within the history of the family lines they belong to and the relationships they maintain with close family over the life course." Influenced by family and occupational events, different generations may live in the same neighbourhood or village or, alternatively, hundreds of kilometres apart. Geographical proximity cannot be considered as an automatic indicator of emotional closeness, however. Indeed, in many cases, distance does not signify a breakdown or weakening of inter-generational ties. On the contrary, it may represent an opportunity to reactivate a relationship (through holiday homes or family homes, Bonvalet and Lelièvre 2005). Similarly, geographical proximity is not always chosen; it may be imposed by circumstance (Bertaux-Wiame 2007).

Before describing the relationships between parents and children in detail, we constructed the geographical map of the network formed by all of the respondent's ascendants, collateral relatives and descendants who are alive at the time of the survey.[7] The average size of the entourage of residents of the Paris region aged

[7] The respondents' parents, adoptive parents, individuals who played a parental role, siblings, current partner and former partners, partners' parents, children and partners' children. Grandchildren are excluded from the calculations.

50–70 at the time of the survey is seven or eight people, with ascendants (the respondent's parents and parents-in-law) accounting for 1.5 people and descendants (the respondent's children and stepchildren) 2 people.

Regarding the spatial distribution of the entourage, we observe that proximity varies with the nature of the relationship (see Table 6.3). Living under the same roof is evidently most frequent with the current partner and children. Beyond the household, geographical proximity takes the following pattern: children live the closest, followed by the respondent's parents and former partners.

Thus, among the respondents who still have a living ascendant, 15 % live in the same or a neighbouring municipality and 13 % live near their parents-in-law. That geographical proximity is important because it adds nuance to the statistics on isolated older persons, which are measured as the number of individuals living alone in their dwelling (Lelièvre and Imbert 2003). The respondents themselves often describe this residential proximity as the ideal solution, resolving many everyday problems faced by older people without the constraints of intergenerational co-residence. It thus preserves everyone's independence for as long as possible.

Unlike the respondents' generation and that of their parents, who experienced massive rural exodus, especially toward Paris, the vast majority of respondents' children did not have to leave their home region to enter the labour force and establish their own households. On the whole, they have left their parents' home recently (at least the children of the 1940–1950 cohorts).

Family support plays an important role in helping adult children find their first accommodation outside their parents' home (Bonvalet 1991). Various family strategies (purchase of a flat, loan of a family-owned home, standing security for a rental property, etc.) are deployed to facilitate young adults' independence. It is often the parents who find their children's first accommodation… close to their own home. Later, the children will be in a position to move further away from their parents, especially when they form their own family and buy their first home.

Table 6.3 Places of residence of members of the family entourage by relationship (%)

Relationship	Co-resident	Same or neighbouring municipality	Total
Parent	1.9	15.3	17.3
Parent-in-law	0.3	13.3	13.6
Adoptive parent	0.0	9.1	9.1
Child	30.5	19.8	50.2
Partner's child	5.2	16.8	22.0
Current partner	89.2	2.0	91.2
Sibling	0.3	11.4	11.7
Former partner	0.7	16.0	16.7
Total	18.8	13.7	32.5

Source: *Biographies et entourage* survey, INED, 2001
Interpretation: 19.8 % of respondents' children were living in the same or a neighbouring municipality at the time of the survey
Coverage: residents of the Paris region born between 1930 and 1950

Owing to the difference in life expectancy between men and women, men are more likely to be living with a partner during retirement (see Table 6.4). The oldest respondents co-reside less frequently with their family because their children have left home. But the spatial distribution of the family network shows that, for one-third (32.5 %) of respondents, regardless of their age, the entourage lives in one of the municipalities neighbouring the respondent's place of residence. The proportion is even higher for residents of the city of Paris (almost four out of ten respondents). And taking the whole kinship network including siblings into account, one-third of respondents have at least one family member living nearby (19 % co-reside and 14 % live in the same or a neighbouring municipality).

Residential proximity is an important factor in the spatial distribution of the family entourage. The residential configuration created by the places of residence of the respondent's ascendants, siblings and descendants is the result of individual trade-offs within the lineage and represents choices or obligations to be close to or distant from family. The territory we observe thus represents the arrangements at a given point in time made to accommodate the specific functioning of each family; it reflects the balance struck between constraints and aspirations within a relationship environment (Bonvalet and Lelièvre 2005).

Although the tendency of families – including siblings – to live close together had already been identified in previous studies (Bonvalet 1991; Gokalp 1978; Roussel 1976; Coenen-Hutter et al. 1994; Attias-Donfut 1996), we are neverthe-

Table 6.4 Places of residence of spatially close members of the family entourage by respondent's characteristics (%)

Respondent's characteristics	Co-resident	Same or neighbouring municipality	Total
Sex			
Male	20.8	13.2	34.0
Female	16.9	14.1	31.0
Cohort			
50–54	21.3	12.7	33.9
55–59	18.0	11.8	29.7
60–64	17.6	15.0	32.6
65+	15.5	17.8	33.3
Area of residence			
Paris	16.7	21.5	38.2
Inner suburbs	19.2	11.6	30.8
Outer suburbs[a]	19.3	13.1	32.4
Satellite towns	19.8	8.4	28.2
All			
	18.8	13.7	32.5

Source: *Biographies et entourage* survey, INED, 2001
Interpretation: 20.8 % of the family entourage (ascendants, partners, children) of male respondents co-reside with the respondent at the time of the survey
Coverage: residents of the Paris region born between 1930 and 1950
[a]Excluding New Towns

less struck by the strong residential proximity of families to their entourage in the most urbanised region of France, where we might have expected families to be more isolated and more disconnected from their kinship networks. While migration to Paris was reflected in uprootedness at the time of the rural exodus, 50 years later families have "put down roots", not only in the city of Paris, but also in the inner and outer suburbs and even in the satellite towns of the Greater Paris region (Imbert 2005).

6.3 Frequency of Contact Between Family Members

The results above provide an initial picture of the family territory of residents of the Paris region aged 50–70. However, they do not tell us anything about the nature of the relationships within that space. Indeed, as we said earlier, residential proximity and distance may result from an occupational constraint (in the case of family businesses for example, Bertaux-Wiame 2007) or from a "family lifestyle". We can analyse relationships within the family more closely by examining affinities and frequency of contact between relatives.

Sociability, particularly in urban areas, has been the focus of many studies by researchers and statisticians (Héran 1988; Bidart 1988; Grafmeyer 1991; Forsé 1993). François Héran, for example, identifies three ages of sociability: "youth is the time of friendships, maturity the time of work relationships, and old age that of kin relationships" (Héran 1988). Sociability within the family holds a particular place: unlike sociability with friends, it does not change with age; contact with kin follows a cycle that revolves around entering and leaving the family group. Initially, when young adults become independent, siblings still play a key role in their relationships. Around age 40–50, the respondents' children and then their children's children broaden the circle, of which they become the centre in their old age.

The respondents therefore hold a double position in the sociability cycle: the youngest respondents, who are still working, have an expanding social network as their children establish their own households and grandchildren are born, while the oldest respondents, who have been retired for some years, are more concentrated on the family.

Frequency of contact between respondents and the members of their entourage was analysed in the *Biographies et entourage* survey on the basis of the responses to the question: "How often are you in contact?". The definition of contact was not restricted to face-to-face meetings.[8]

[8] The interviewers were instructed to specify that contact could be by telephone, in writing or by other means. We therefore do not know whether contact was face-to-face or not. The open questions were coded ex-post to prevent respondents from standardizing their responses by conforming to the analysis categories.

6.3.1 Relationships Between Respondents and Their Parents

The interviews from *Biographies et entourage* conducted after the quantitative survey show that closeness or distance between parents and children depend on the individuals' personalities, marital status and family history. We were thus able, for each respondent, to reconstruct the meaning of moves in the light of his/her social trajectory. However, we initially took a purely statistical, descriptive approach to identify the main trends in these proximities. The snapshot that the survey provides is the result of the "geographical and emotional" distances that play out between parents and children over a lifetime, in response to occupational trajectories and demographic events.

At the time of the survey, half of the respondents (49 %) are in contact with their parent(s) at least once a week. But there are strong disparities, with 13 % of respondents being in daily contact and 9 % having no contact. On average, respondents are in contact with their parents twice-weekly.

When both of the respondent's parents are still alive, four-fifths reported the same frequency of contact with both parents. Of the remaining one-fifth, 78 % reported more frequent contact with their mother than with their father. That result can be partly attributed to separated parents, and partly to the fact that respondents speak more often with their mothers (e.g. on the telephone), even when both parents are still living together.[9]

We next refined the analysis by considering the responses to the question: "How many people do you feel close to and who are they?". We found only a small difference between the percentages of (living) fathers and mothers considered close: 51 % of respondents whose mother is alive consider her close, and 44 % say the same of their fathers.

A similar analysis was conducted on the *Proches et parents* survey and showed that the degree of affinity with parents does not change with the respondent's age, but that it does with the parent's age, which determines the nature of the relationship. There is less closeness when mothers are aged over 75. That result is particularly surprising as geographical proximity increases with age. Although the ageing of parents may cause the generations to move geographically closer, this does not reflect a strengthening of affinities. "In fact, the dynamic of the relationship changes and, after a certain age, elderly parents are mainly perceived as needing care. This encourages us to think that the concept of closeness refers to a degree of mutual exchange, to a relationship that is not too dissymmetrical" (Bonvalet and Maison 2007).

Women – both female respondents and the mothers of respondents – are in contact with their ascendant(s) and descendant(s) more frequently than men. All other things being equal, men are less likely than women to be in weekly contact with their parent(s) (see Table 6.5).

[9] Consequently, in our analysis, the frequency of contact with the mother was used for respondents who reported a different relationship with their father and mother (approximately 50 respondents).

Table 6.5 Distribution of respondents in contact with their parent(s) at least once a week

By sex	%
Respondent...	
... is a woman	53
... is a man	44
... has only mother alive	53
... has only father alive	33
... has both parents alive	48
By entourage composition	
Respondent...	
... lives with a partner	48
... does not live with a partner	55
Parents' entourage comprises...	
... 0–2 people	47
... 2–4 people	59
... 4–6 people	44
... 6 or more people	33
Total	**49**

We thus confirm a well-known result: it is usually the women in the family who organize kinship relationships, sometimes replacing their partner. "They appear clearly as the primary artisans of family relationships and exchanges" (Hammer et al. 2001).

A higher proportion of respondents who do not live in a couple are in contact with their parent(s) at least weekly than of respondents who live with a partner (see Table 6.5). Aside from the presence or absence of a partner, the respondent's entourage influences the frequency of contact with his/her parent(s).

If we include in the respondent's entourage all his/her siblings, all of his/her partner's siblings, his/her parents and parents-in-law, and his/her children, it consists of seven or eight people on average, as we saw earlier.

Respondents whose entourage consists of fewer than 5 people are in contact with their parent(s) almost twice weekly, which is twice as often as respondents whose entourage includes 10–15 people.[10]

In terms of the composition of the entourage, frequency of contact is not influenced by the number of the respondent's children or whether the respondent's in-laws are still alive, but rather by the number of the respondent's siblings. Reciprocally, for the parents, being in a couple and the number of children (including the respondent) play a significant role.

The larger the parents' entourage, the lower the frequency of contact with the respondent. When the parents' entourage consists of two to four people, the

[10] When the respondent has a large entourage, the probability that he/she is the child in most frequent contact with the parents is lower than when the respondent has a small entourage.

respondent has more opportunity to be in weekly contact than when the parents have a larger entourage (four to six people).

This implies that the attention given to parent(s) is shared between their children, which confirms the practice of a division of roles between siblings toward their elderly parents, especially when one of the siblings is single and childless. That sibling, more attached to the parents because he/she has not formed his/her own family, is in an easier position to maintain a close relationship with the elderly parent.[11]

Unfortunately, we do not have any information about the frequency of contact of each sibling. Consequently, we cannot compare the different frequencies of contact with the same parent by all of his/her children.

6.3.2 Relationships between Respondents Living with a Partner and Their Ascendants

When respondents living in a couple at the time of the survey[12] are asked about the frequency of contact with their parents and parents-in-law, they report talking more often to mothers and mothers-in-law than to fathers and fathers-in-law. The results in Table 6.6 describe the frequency of contact with parents, but comparing different percentages is not easy. Moreover, if we compare a respondent's different statements about each of his/her ascendants, we will be measuring affinities or dislikes, and not necessarily the couple's socialization with their ascendants.

We therefore examined the distances between the places of residence of the parents and parents-in-law among respondents with at least one living parent and one living in-law (27 % of the respondents in a couple, 21 % of respondents living in the Paris region aged 50–70). Some 40 % of them live very near to their parents and 33 % very near to their parents-in-law. No significant difference appears between the families of the woman or the man. This low percentage is probably due to the Paris region where many respondents of these generations settled from other places, which blurs the map of spatial proximity with parents.

[11] Co-residence, i.e. when the respondent lives under the same roof as his/her father or mother, is rare; it concerns 2.4 % of living parents. In most of these cases, the parent (usually the mother) no longer has a partner. Respondents who co-reside with their parent(s) may accommodate them or be accommodated by them, and in 60 % of cases are themselves separated or widowed. An overrepresentation of manual workers skews the results, both in terms of the respondents (28 % of co-resident respondents were manual workers) and parents (47 % of fathers or partners of co-resident mothers were manual workers). The proportions appear to be smaller for the total population.

[12] They represent three-quarters of the sample.

Table 6.6 Proportion (%) of respondents in contact with their parent(s) at least once a week[a]

	Mother	Mother-in-law	Father	Father-in-law
Female respondents	55	15	43	18
Male respondents	45	30	32	28
Number of respondents with a living parent	*922*	*424*	*426*	*558*

Source: *Biographies et entourage* survey, INED, 2001
Coverage: residents of Greater Paris born between 1930 and 1950
[a]Multiple responses are allowed

6.3.3 Relationships between Respondents Aged over 60 and Their Children

For respondents aged over 60 with one child living outside the household, 70 % are in at least weekly contact with that child. If the child is a daughter, the frequency increases: three-quarters are in contact at least once a week.

If we consider the case of respondents with two children living independently, when the children are of the same sex, a higher percentage of respondents say they are in contact with both children equally frequently. When the children are of different sexes, 12 % report being in contact at least once a week with their daughter and less frequently with their son. Conversely, only 5 % say they contact their son more often. However, one-quarter of respondents report being in contact with both daughter and son at least once a week.

6.4 Frequency of Contact and Residential Proximity of Family Members

The *Biographies et entourage* survey data can be used to examine the frequency of contact – face-to-face meetings, telephone calls and electronic communication – with parents, and to cross-reference this information with geographical distance, measured here by the number of kilometres between the respondent's place of residence and their parent's/parents' home. We thus combine the two indicators. Given that the question was not restricted to face-to-face meetings and that the family's spatial distribution is uneven, how does geographical distance interact with emotional closeness?

Proximity between parents' and children's places of residence has a decisive influence on their relationship by facilitating daily or weekly contact: 38 % of respondents who live less than 10 km from a parent are in daily contact, compared with 5 % of respondents who live 200–500 km from a parent. A higher frequency of contact (telephone calls, visits, letters) is much easier when the respondent and his/her parent(s) live close to each other.

However, when contact between respondents and their parents is less frequent than weekly, distance no longer seems to have a major influence. Figure 6.3 shows only three curves (for the sake of clarity), which correspond to thresholds of

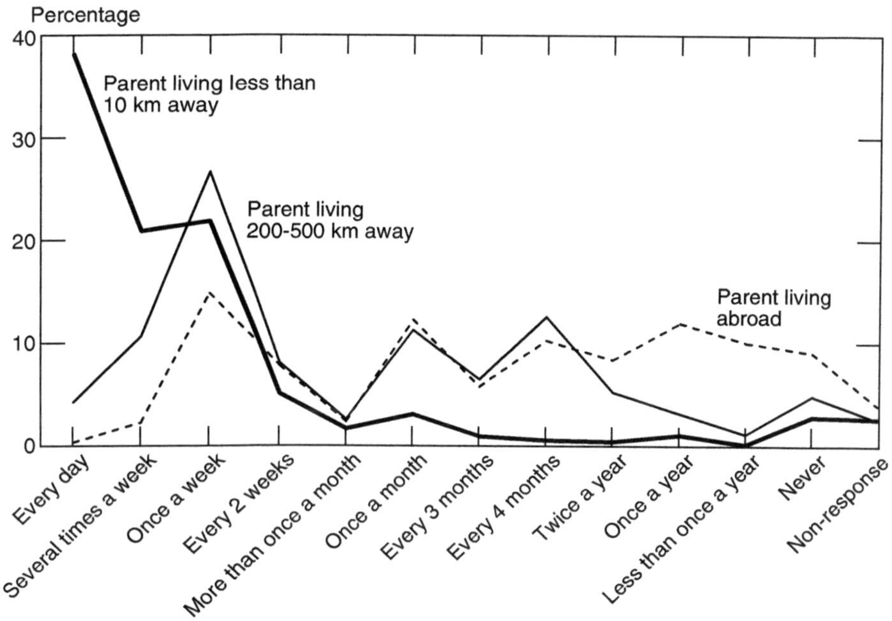

Fig. 6.3 Frequency of contact and residential distance between respondents and their parent(s) (*Source*: *Biographies et entourage* survey, INED, 2001)

distances between the respondent's home and that of his/her parents: less than 10 km; 200–500 km; and abroad. The percentage of respondents who report contact every 2 weeks, every month or every 4 months is the same for respondents whose parents live 200–500 km away or abroad.

6.4.1 *The Generations Move Closer as Parents Enter Old Age*

At the time of the survey, 36 % of the 2830 respondents intended to move home, compared with 63 % who intended to remain in their current home. A majority of residents of the Paris region aged 50–70 thus expressed an intention of stability.

For one-third of residents of the Paris region who want to move home (who tend to be younger and still working), the reasons for wishing to move are related to the comfort of their dwelling (33 % of respondents) or their neighbourhood (30 %). Next come considerations relating to the environment and the climate (9 %), financial problems (9 %) and a wish to return to their region or country of origin (8 %).

A wish to be close to children is cited as a reason both by those who intend to move and those who intend to remain in their current home. This reason is most commonly given by the cohorts born before 1940. Some 14 % of respondents aged over 60 wish to stay in their current home so that they stay near their children (compared with 7 % of the younger cohorts).

6.5 Conclusion

Based on three indicators (emotional closeness, geographical distance, and frequency of contact), we attempted to capture the family environment of older people. These indicators correspond to three of the six conceptual dimensions of the micro-social model of intergenerational solidarity developed by Bengtson in the 1970s (Bengtson et al. 1976; Bengtson and Roberts 1991), namely affectual solidarity, structural solidarity (co-residence and geographical proximity) and associational solidarity (frequency of contact). The *Biographies et entourage* survey data do not enable us to study functional solidarity (giving and receiving of support), consensual solidarity (agreement in opinions) or normative solidarity (agreement on family values), however our analysis of the survey data confirms that the cohorts aged 50–70 are strongly involved in their family networks. They thus play their role as the "sandwich generation" between their elderly parents and their children. These cohorts have experienced the family transition from a model where relationships of authority and supremacy of the group predominated, to the model of the "chosen" family, where the quality of relationships takes precedence over their hierarchy. While, in their youth, some of this generation would have identified with books like *Finie la famille ?* and *The Death of the Family* that emphasized the importance of the couple over the family (de Singly 1993, 1994) and initiated new family behaviours (non-marital cohabitation, divorce), the vast majority were able, in their maturity, to develop different relationships both with their parents and with their children and grandchildren, to the point where some researchers have seen the emergence of "new grandparents" (Attias-Donfut and Segalen 1998) and a "new family spirit" (Attias-Donfut et al. 2002). But this transformation is not so overarching as to affect the continuity of family relationships, as reflected in the respondents' accounts of their relationships with their own grandparents, despite the breakdown of relationships that has occurred in some families.

Appendix

Table A.1 Proportion of living parents by respondents' age (%)

	Respondents aged under 60	Respondents aged over 60	Total respondents (aged 50–70)
No living ascendant	40	76	54
1 living ascendant	40	20	32
2 living ascendants	20	4	14
Total	100	100	100

Source: *Biographies et entourage* survey, INED, 2001
Coverage: residents of Paris region born between 1930 and 1950

Table A.2 Proportion of living ascendants (parents and parents-in-law) by respondent's age (%)

	At least one of the two partners is under 60	Both partners are over 60	Respondents living with a partner
No living ascendant	19	55	29
1 living ascendant	32	28	31
2 living ascendants	28	13	24
3 living ascendants	15	3	12
4 living ascendants	6	–	4
Total	100	100	100

Source: *Biographies et entourage* survey, INED, 2001
Coverage: residents of Paris region born between 1930 and 1950

References

Attias-Donfut, C. (Ed.). (1995). *Les solidarités entre générations: vieillesse, familles, État*. Paris: Nathan.

Attias-Donfut, C. (1996). Les solidarités centre générations. In *Données sociales* (pp. 317–323). Paris: INSEE

Attias-Donfut, C., & Segalen, M. (1998). *Grands-parents: la famille à travers les générations*. Paris: Odile Jacob.

Attias-Donfut, O., Segalen, M., & Lapierre, N. (2002). *Le nouvel esprit de famille*. Paris: Odile Jacob.

Bengtson, V. L., & Roberts, R. E. L. (1991). Intergenerational solidarity in aging families: An example of formal theory construction. *Journal of Marriage and the Family, 53*, 856–870.

Bengtson, V. L., Olander, E. B., & Haddad, A. A. (1976). The 'génération gap' and aging family members: Toward a conceptual model. In J. F. Cubrium (Ed.), *Time, roles and self in old age*. New York: Human Sciences Press.

Bertaux-Wiame, I. (2007). Work, home and family: An analysis of several residential configurations of persons with independent occupations. In C. Bonvalet, A. Gotman, & Y. Grafmeyer (Eds.), *Family, kinship and place in France* (pp. 181–202). London: Southern Universities Press.

Bidart, C. (1988). Sociabilités : quelques variables. *Revue française de sociologie, 29*, 621–648.

Bonvalet, C. (1991). La famille et le marché du logement : une logique cachée ? In M. Segalen (Ed.), *Jeux de familles* (pp. 57–77). Paris: CNRS Éditions.

Bonvalet, C. (2003). The local family circle. *Population, English Edition, 58*(1), 9–42.

Bonvalet, C., & Lelièvre, É. (1995). Du concept de ménage à celui d'entourage : une redéfinition de l'espace familial. *Sociologie et societes, 27*(2), 177–190.

Bonvalet, C., & Lelièvre, É. (2005). Les lieux de la famille. *Espaces et sociétés, La famille dans tous ses espaces, 1–2*(2005), 99–122.

Bonvalet, C., & Maison, D. (2007). The family circle: Spatial proximity and personal affinity. In C. Bonvalet, A. Gotman, & Y. Grafmeyer (Eds.), *Family, kinship and place in France* (pp. 27–68). London: Southern Universities Press.

Bonvalet, C., Maison, D., Le Bras, H., & Charles, L. (1993). Proches et parents. *Population, 48*(1), 83–110.

Coenen-Hutter, J., Kellerhals, J., & Von Allmen, M. (1994). *Les réseaux de solidarité dans la famille*. Lausanne: Éditions Réalités sociales.

Collectif. (1975). *Finie la famille ? Traditions et nouveaux rôles* (n°3, 191 p.). Paris: Autrement.

Cooper, D. (1970). *The death of the family*. New York: Pantheon Books. 145 p.

Crenner, E. (1998). La parenté : un réseau de sociabilité actif mais concentré. *Insee Première*, 600.

de Singly, F. (1993). Comment définir la famille contemporaine ? *Études statistiques, 4*, 31–39.

de Singly, F. (1994). *Sociologie de la famille contemporaine*. Paris: Nathan.
Delbès, C., & Gaymu, J. (2003). More unions surviving after 60? *Population and Societies,* INED, 389.
Désesquelles, A., & Brouard, N. (2003). The family networks of people aged 60 and over living at home or in an institution. *Population, 58*(2), 181–206.
Forsé, M. (1993). La fréquence des relations de sociabilité : typologie et évolutions. *L'Année sociologique, 43*, 189–212.
Gokalp, C. (1978). Le réseau familial. *Population, 33*(6), 1077–1094.
Gotman, A. (2007). Family geographies, migrations and generations. In C. Bonvalet, A. Gotman, & Y. Grafmeyer (Eds.), *Family, kinship and place in France* (pp. 69–133). London: Southern Universities Press.
Grafmeyer, Y. (1991). *Habiter Lyon. Milieux et quartiers du centre-ville*. Paris/Lyon: Éditions du CNRS/Presses universitaires de Lyon/PPSH.
Guillemard, A.-M. (Ed.). (1991). *La retraite en mutation,* rapport Centre d'étude des mouvements sociaux. Paris: FEN.
Hammer, R., Burton-Jeangros, C., & Kellerhals, J. (2001). Le lien de parenté dans les Jeunes générations suisses : lignées, structure et fonctions. *Population, 56*(4), 515–537.
Héran, F. (1988). La sociabilité, une pratique culturelle. *Économie et Statistique, 216*, 3–22.
Imbert, C. (2005). Ancrage et proximités familiales dans les villes nouvelles franciliennes : une approche comparative. *Espaces et sociétés, 119*, 159–176.
Le Bras, H., & Roussel, L. (1982). Retard ou refus du mariage : l'évolution récente de la première nuptialité en France et sa prévision. *Population, 37*(6), 1009–1044.
Lelièvre, É., & Imbert, C. (2003). L'entourage des Franciliens de 50 à 70 ans s'étend au-delà des limites de la région. In Iaurif, *Atlas des Franciliens* (Vol. 3, pp. 44–45). Paris, INSEE.
Lelièvre, É., & Vivier, G. (2001). Évaluation d'une collecte à la croisée du quantitatif et du qualitatif, l'enquête *Biographies et entourage. Population, 56*(6), 1043–1074.
Lelièvre, É., Bonvalet, C., & Bry, X. (1998). Event history analysis of groups. The findings of an on-going research project. *Population, an English Selection, 10*(1), 11–37.
Monnier, A., & Pennec, S. (2003). Three per cent of under-21s are parentless in France. *Population and Societies,* INED, 396.
Roussel, L. (1976). La famille après le mariage des enfants : les relations entre générations. *Population, 31*(6), 1195–1206.
Young, M., & Willmott, P. (1957). *Family and kinship in East London*. London: Routledge and Kegan Paul.

Chapter 7
Grandparents: From Neglect to Idolization

Catherine Bonvalet and Éva Lelièvre

Grandparents are the custodians of memories – family memories, but also memories of the last century of history. Their narratives of events large and small that have marked their country, their city, their village, and therefore also their close circle of family and friends, represent a link between past and future generations. Grandparents play a central role in passing on family memories, without which personal identities could not be constructed, as grandparents are the "privileged figures upon whom this existential desire to be part of a succession through time is projected" (Gourdon 2001, p. 351).

And yet, in France, all researchers, whether historians or sociologists, are in agreement about the limited corpus of work on grandparents that characterized research on the family up to the late 1980s. Louis Roussel (1976), Catherine Gokalp (1978), and Agnès Pitrou (1978) stood out as pioneers. In the 1990s, with the crisis in the welfare state, the declining influence of ideologies and the rise in social disadvantage, a resurgence of interest in family-based forms of solidarity was observed. Major surveys[1] were undertaken by INSEE (the French National Institute for Statistics and Economic Studies), INED (the French Institute for Demographic Studies) and CNAV (the French National Retirement Insurance Fund). With the rise of divorce and separation, the nuclear family, which had been the modern reference for family life in the two decades following the Second World War, in opposition to the traditional rural family, began to weaken its hold, with the result that ties of affinity faded in favour of blood ties. Kinship became the keystone of the family

This chapter was first published in French in *Mémoire et démographie, regards croisés au Sud et au Nord*, Richard Marcoux and J. Dion (eds.), 2009, Québec, Presses de l'Université Laval, coll. "Cahiers du CIEQ", pp. 260–270.

[1] INSEE, *Enquête sur les réseaux de sociabilité* (1990); INED, *Proches et parents* survey (1990); CNAV, *Trois generations* survey (1992).

C. Bonvalet (✉) • É. Lelièvre (✉)
Institut national d'études démographiques (INED), Paris, France
e-mail: bonvalet@ined.fr; eva@ined.fr

C. Bonvalet, É. Lelièvre (eds.), *Family Beyond Household and Kin*,
INED Population Studies 6, DOI 10.1007/978-3-319-24684-0_7

system, and a place of solidarity and protection, while the couple was transformed into a place of negotiation. In the French academic field of history, before the 1991 special edition of *Annales de démographie historique*[2] and above all Vincent Gourdon's PhD thesis (2001) on the history of grandparents, there existed no research on grandparenthood from the *Ancien Régime* to the present day that clearly highlighted the indisputably important role played by grandparents in the societies of yesteryear.

The hypothesis we explore in this chapter – which follows in the footsteps of Vincent Gourdon's work – is that French researchers show signs of amnesia when they talk about new discoveries with regard to grandparents. The history of the sociology of the family is marked by the recurrent assertion that new family forms have emerged: conjugal families, single-parent families, stepfamilies – and now the new extended family? Why must we talk about *new family spirit* in order to restore the image of the extended family? Is it to avoid harking back to a traditional concept, and thereby show proof of modernity?

This work, in which memories are of great importance, takes as its starting point the *Biographies et entourage* survey, conducted by INED with the aim of retracing the family history of cohorts born between 1930 and 1950. On the one hand, the quantitative data can be used to analyse the parental role played by respondents' grandparents; on the other, qualitative interviews enable us to establish the extent to which these grandparents have influenced the construction of respondents' identities, and how their memories of their grandparents have influenced they way they act as grandparents themselves.

7.1 The Vision of the Family Since the Nineteenth Century: A Scientific Memory

Since the nineteenth century, the family has generated a great deal of research. As Cicchelli-Pugeault and Cicchelli (1998) explain, Tocqueville was among the first to develop a sociology of family relationships. In his view, the weakening of intergenerational relationships characterized the family in America and in particular the decline of lineage: "the family no longer enters the mind except as something vague, indeterminate and uncertain" (1835). A few years later, Auguste Comte referred to the model of mediaeval chivalry to define the role of the family in maintaining social links. In his view, the family, "the unmistakeable basis of society", must

[2] The 1991 issue of *Annales de démographie historique*, devoted to grandparents and elders, includes an article on the art of being a grandmother in the seventeenth, eighteenth and nineteenth centuries (by Jean-Pierre Bois, 1991), as well as an article on yesterday's grandfathers, also from the seventeenth to the nineteenth centuries (by Madeleine Foisil, 1991), in which a number of models – in particular the grandfather in the context of family continuity, the grandfather in and of himself, and the made-to-measure grandfather – are presented.

constitute a "protectorate" for its weakest members (Comte 1995 [1839]). In France, another precursor in the field was without doubt Le Play, although his work was criticized by Durkheim: "In yesterday's families, some will seek models to propose for our imitation" (1888). Durkheim picked up where Tocqueville left off (although he never explicitly acknowledged this fact), and similarly observed changes in the family: "There is nothing left that recalls this state of perpetual dependence which was the basis of the paternal family" (1871). In the contemporary family, the intergenerational dimension no longer structures family relationships. "This is why the conjugal family, which is too ephemeral since it dissolves with death in every generation, cannot guarantee the maintenance of social ties" (1892). But it is the theories of sociologist Talcott Parsons that have had the greatest influence on the theme of mutual family support. Like Engels, Marx, Tocqueville, Comte and Durkheim (1975), "who treat domestic organization as a dependent variable of social structure", Parsons maintains that the family institution was transformed by the Industrial Revolution (1998). Parsons' theory, developed in the 1930s, only truly began to gain momentum in the 1950s. Taking as his starting point the notion of the "private nuclear family", the dominant family structure that emerged in the Western world after industrialization, Parsons evoked the inevitable trend towards the uniformity of this structure in modern societies. The nuclear family, created by marriage, lives in a separate dwelling from the extended family and lives on its own economic resources, thanks to income from the husband's job, "independently of any particularistic relation to kinsmen" (1943). Following on from Tocqueville and Comte, Parsons advocates the division of tasks within the household – economic for the husband and domestic for the wife – to ensure that the family functions with the greatest possible efficiency.

It is in part because these authors focused on the structure of the household that they somewhat overlooked the family, and consequently deduced a weakening of kinship links and a reduction in mutual support, as pointed out by the historians Burguière and Stone (Burguière et al. 1986; Stone 1977). Parsons' theory has generated a number of controversies and given rise to a whole new series of surveys, the "family history" of which we retraced in a book (Bonvalet and Ogg 2007). Indeed, over the last two decades or so, research into the extended family has grown and major surveys have been conducted on the subject of relationships and exchanges in the context of kinship in France and Europe.

In parallel, there are many studies in the sociology of the family concerning couples with children, single-parent families or stepfamilies – i.e. concerning family groups resulting from co-residence. The notions put forward to describe the contemporary family are those of individualization, independence and the creation of a certain distance with regard to kin – in other words, a movement away from the close-knit family circle (de Singly 1991, 1993a, 1993b). There is therefore an opposition between research that focuses on the couple and research into the extended family. With this in mind, Florence Weber suggested returning to the concepts of household and kin group since "thinking about family relationships today without the help of the tools provided by the anthropology of kinship leads to inaccuracies and even confusion" (Weber 2002, p. 73). For his part, François de Singly (1993a, p. 68) attempted to reconcile this opposition, writing that "the misunderstandings [...] that exist in the sociology of the family concerning the role of family and kinship in contemporary societies arise from the fact that specialists construct their reasoning on the basis of an 'either/or' alternative". On the other hand, while the rise in divorce is tending to weaken conjugal relations, Irène Théry pointed out that "the filial relation is increasingly asserted as an unconditional" and indissoluble relationship (1995, p. 106) that forms part of the long-term structure of family ties. Accordingly, she identified "two contrasting movements at the origin of transformations in the contemporary family [...]; one functions in the sense of a contractual link [*conjugal*], and the other in the sense of an unconditionality [*of the filial link*]" (1998, p. 38). She stressed that "the effects of the fragility of couples on filial relations has become a major social issue" (1998, p. 49).

And yet it would seem that new misunderstandings still exist around kinship, especially regarding grandparents. Researchers working on these themes have experienced the transition of the family – i.e. the transition from a family where relations of authority and the supremacy of the group (where the individual serves the interests of the family) tended to dominate, to the "chosen" family, in which the quality of the relationship is more important than its nature. While a number of these researchers, in their youth, made contributions to the works *Finie la famille* ? (Collectif 1975) and *Mort de la famille* (Cooper 1972), which asserted the supremacy of the couple over kinship (de Singly 1993a), and, along with the rest of their generation, were the initiators of new family behaviours (cohabitation outside marriage, divorce), they have "rediscovered the family" to such an extent that some authors talk about "new grandparents" (Attias-Donfut and Segalen 1998) or "new family spirit" (Attias-Donfut et al. 2002).

7.2 Yesterday's Grandparents and Today's Grandparents

It would seem, therefore, that grandparents currently occupy a central role in the family, so much so that sociologists talk about "new-style" grandparents: "there are many characteristics that point to the modernity of grandparents' style. A revival of ties, more communication between generations, a liberation in terms of expressing love and affection, a more informal and playful relationship" (Attias-Donfut and Segalen 1998). This vision of the "cake-baking" grandparent perpetuates, "more often than not, a truncated or imagined vision of the history of grandparents" (Gourdon 2001, p. 102). According to Vincent Gourdon, the image of the cake-baking grandparent came into being in the nineteenth century with the rise of bourgeois family values (*L'Art d'être grand-père* by Victor Hugo). Not only were grandparents present in the eighteenth and nineteenth centuries, but they were also already playing a role that complemented that of the parents.

Indeed, in the mid-eighteenth century, contrary to popular belief, grandparents had their place in society.[3] Furthermore, according to Le Bras's calculations (1973, p. 27), in the eighteenth century, just 16 % of children had no grandparents at birth, with the proportion rising to 38 % at age 10 and 73 % at age 21. The majority of children therefore knew at least one grandparent during childhood.

7.3 Grandparents: What Data Are Available?

The empirical material with which we have worked here is partly quantitative and partly composed of qualitative interviews. INED's *Biographies et entourage* survey traces the family, residential and occupational history of each respondent and his or her entourage. This entourage, made up of different family members (blood relatives and affines) from four generations, also includes all persons with whom the individual has co-resided since birth and other people who, whether related or not, have played a key role in the respondents' lives. The extension of data collection from the individual to members of the "entourage" seeks to place the individual within his or her sphere of influence in order to enrich the analysis of individual trajectories using information collected about close friends and family, and gauge the impact of this entourage on individual trajectories. This approach therefore combines individual trajectories, personal networks of influence and the societal environment in a long-term perspective (Lelièvre and Vivier 2001).

Regarding grandparenthood, the survey data allow to combine three perspectives within each descent group: respondents' relationships with their grandparents, especially during childhood, which in the case of our sample population occurred between the 1930s the 1960s; the relationships of respondents' children with respondents' parents; and lastly, respondents' relationships as grandparents with their grandchildren.

The interviews used here were conducted as part of explorations that sought to clarify the way in which intergenerational relationships function within the entourage. This long-term project brings together interviews collected since the early 1990s resulting from return visits to respondents from the *Proches et parents* and *Biographies et entourage* surveys. Here, we have selected – on a thematic basis following a conventional content analysis – those that more specifically evoke interactions with grandparents (both with their own grandparents and as grandparents themselves). Regarding those grandparents cited as having played a parental role by respondents in *Biographies and entourage*, we have also used a textual analysis of free-form responses describing these roles in detail.

In this chapter, we consider respondents as "interlocutors" and, more specifically, explore their relationships with their own grandparents; we address the opposite situation (i.e. the respondents as grandparents) more succinctly. The combination of

[3] Regarding the situation in England, see the latest works by Steven Ruggles on the nineteenth century, the works of Laslett, and the works of Young and Willmott (1957).

quantitative data and interviews gives us a better understanding of the place and role of grandparents for respondents from cohorts born between 1930 and 1950, and whose grandparents were therefore born in the late nineteenth and early twentieth centuries.

During childhood or adolescence, more than a quarter of respondents (25.6 %) reported having lived for at least a year with a grandparent, with a third (32 %) reporting that their grandparents resided in the same municipality or in an adjacent municipality. Another indicator available to us is whether or not respondents regularly spent time at their grandparents' home during the holidays, weekends, evenings after school, etc., which was the case for one respondent in five (19.3 %). However, some respondents may, for instance, have both lived with their grandmother for a while and lived nearby later, or lived with their paternal grandmother while remaining in close geographical proximity to their maternal grandparents, since each respondent has two pairs of grandparents who are not distinguished in the survey. The proportion of respondents who lived with or near their grandparents during childhood and adolescence is therefore probably around half – and this proportion grows with successive birth cohorts and increasing life expectancies.

Although we cannot accurately measure how these situations overlap, we can nevertheless give an approximate proportion of respondents who have lived in a family environment where their grandparents were relatively absent: this figure stands at around 40 %.

Overall, therefore, grandparents have been very much present in respondents' lives. To further explore the nature of the relationship between respondents and their grandparents, we shall now focus on those respondents who reported in the *Biographies et entourage* survey that their grandparents had played a parental role.

7.4 Yesterday's Grandparents

The *Biographies et entourage* survey involved collecting data relating to milestones in the family, occupational and residential histories of respondents and of members of their entourage, situating these individuals within their networks and their spheres of influence. These spheres were identified by collecting of information on the trajectories of individuals in respondents' entourage, whether family members (blood relatives, collateral relatives, affines), friends, co-residents, or other people cited as having played a key role in their lives.

With respect to respondents' childhoods, the care taken in constructing the questionnaire and in identifying the collection categories which made sense for the respondents led to unexpected figures being uncovered in the childhood sphere – individuals reported by respondents as having played a parental role for them who were neither their father or their mother, or who were not even family members in some cases (Lelièvre and Vivier 2001). When asked about other people who had

Table 7.1 Distribution of parental roles according to kinship ties with respondents (%)

Kinship tie with respondent	
Within the family realm	
Grandparents	51
Aunt or uncle	20
Brother or sister	8
Other relatives	5
Outside the family realm	
Contractual link with parents	7
Other unrelated person	9
Total %	100
Total population	803

Source: *Biographies et entourage* survey, INED, 2001

had a significant positive or negative influence at different stages of their lives (childhood, adolescence, young adulthood, etc.),[4] some respondents also mentioned other reference figures in their youth, notably people with an educational role.

In all, 585 respondents, or one in five, mentioned the presence of at least one other parental figure in childhood (Lelièvre et al. 2008); in total, therefore, 803 individuals were cited as having played a parental role in childhood for 20 % of our population of respondents. These individuals were mainly family members, and more than half were grandparents (Table 7.1), essentially female (67 % female and 33 % male), although 16 % of those cited had no kinship ties with respondents. In the current context, where the involvement and the "new role" of grandparents with regard to their grandchildren is often highlighted, it is important to emphasize that these alternative or additional parental figures were grandfathers or grandmothers in half of all cases.

Respondents who reported the involvement of elective parent figures in their childhood usually cite only one person, generally a woman (in 79 % of cases where only one additional figure was cited) and, more often than not, a grandmother, whose presence is therefore quite remarkable.

Those respondents who mentioned more than one individual most often referred to couples (in 60 % of cases). Typically, these couples were respondents' maternal or paternal grandparents. Accordingly, grandparents – highly present in their grandchildren's lives – account for the majority of the couples cited. They therefore contributed significantly to shaping the family life and upbringing of these respondents born between 1930 and 1950. Few respondents cited more than two individuals.

[4] The question that was asked, namely "Apart from these individuals, are there any others – friends, family members and in-laws, colleagues, etc. – who have been or who are important to you, positively or negatively?", aimed to avoid restricting the entourage to the family sphere, so that other circles of sociability and influence, such as networks of friends or colleagues, neighbours, etc. could be included.

Table 7.2 Distribution of parental roles by place of residence during the period in which this role was assumed (%)

Link with respondent	Place of residence (with respect to the respondent)				
	Co-resident	Immediate vicinity	Elsewhere	Total %	Total population
Within the family realm					
Grandparents	72	16	12	100	403
Brother or sister	72	12	16	100	52
Aunt/uncle, other relatives	51	27	22	100	221
Outside the family realm					
Contractual link, foster family	85	6	9	100	79
Friend, god parent	26	44	30	100	48
All parental roles	65	20	16	100	803

Source: *Biographies et entourage* survey, INED, 2001

7.4.1 Co-residence and Geographical Proximity

In residential terms, the contexts of these relationships are marked by the fact that the individuals assuming parental roles lived in the same municipality as the respondent (or a neighbouring municipality), and very frequently in the same dwelling (Table 7.2).

Overall, 65 % of individuals in "parental roles" lived with the respondent at some point. In cases of co-residence, these individuals were grandparents in the majority of cases, be it in the respondent's home or in their own home. For another quarter of these individuals, this role was taken on without necessarily sharing the respondent's daily living space.

7.4.2 The Specific Role of Grandmothers

The quantitative questionnaire for *Biographies et entourage* contained three modules that collected details of the trajectories of (1) biological parents, (2) adoptive parents and (3) the spouses of these parents, followed by a section exploring the existence of other individuals who played a parental role in respondents' lives. If any such individuals were cited, respondents were invited to complete a free-form description of the nature of the influence exerted by the persons in question. A textual analysis of the roles played by these individuals then made it possible to specify not just the functions they fulfilled, but also some of their characteristics (Chap. 4).

In general, when asked the question, "In what way has this person played a parental role for you?", respondents answer in terms of the functions this person performed and the circumstances of the parental influence exercised, and personal characteristics. Respondents first gave their reason for citing a given parental figure by explaining the functions that this individual performed for them. These reasons can be divided into four broad categories, namely (in order of frequency) material tasks (*feeding, nursing, supporting, looking after, caring for, taking care of*, etc.), tasks relating to stimulation, socialization and education (*teaching things, contributing*, etc.), emotional and psychological roles (*loving, cherishing, acting as a role model, admiring*, etc.), and lastly the exercise of responsibility and authority. Next, respondents provided information explaining the context of their involvement, specifying the historical or family circumstances that led to this individual taking on a parental role. Finally, they gave "descriptive" elements characterizing the personality or status (social, professional, etc.) of the individual concerned.

Grandmothers – the most frequently cited parent figures – were characterized by the diversity of functions assigned to them in material terms (using words such as: *housekeeper, support, ingredient, kitchen, prepare, care, contagious*) and in psychological and intellectual terms (*share, cheerful, museums, teach things, available*).

Grandmothers were the figures most often cited as compensating for the absence of a mother. Their emotional and psychological roles were often mentioned in counterpoint to a mother who was less available.

> While my mother was giving sewing lessons, she did the cooking, looked after us, she was the woman of the house. She was a very affectionate grandmother, it was she who raised us, a second mother… when she died, I was so sad that I became ill. My grandmother filled in for my sick mother. [She] looked after the house, took care of everything and was a figure of authority. She educated me. I would sleep in her bedroom.[5]

Grandmothers were above all cited in the context of everyday life. In addition, respondents' relationships with their grandmothers form part of a wider female family culture and heritage (female respondents cited their grandmothers more often than men) and strongly depend on the relationship between (female) respondents and their own mothers. Analyses of in-depth interviews confirmed this observation and extended these findings by examining this familial transmission in greater detail.

7.4.3 Entrusted to Others

Of the 2,830 respondents, a quarter had lived for a time without their parents before the age of 15 (the age at which compulsory education ended and apprenticeships began for these cohorts born between 1930 and 1950). For 40 % of them, it was a time spent in boarding school, while 6 % had already embarked upon an apprenticeship. However, more than half (52 %) of those who grew up without their parents were entrusted to third parties (Lelièvre et al. 2008).

---

[5] Excerpts from the open questions in the *Biographies et entourage* quantitative questionnaire.

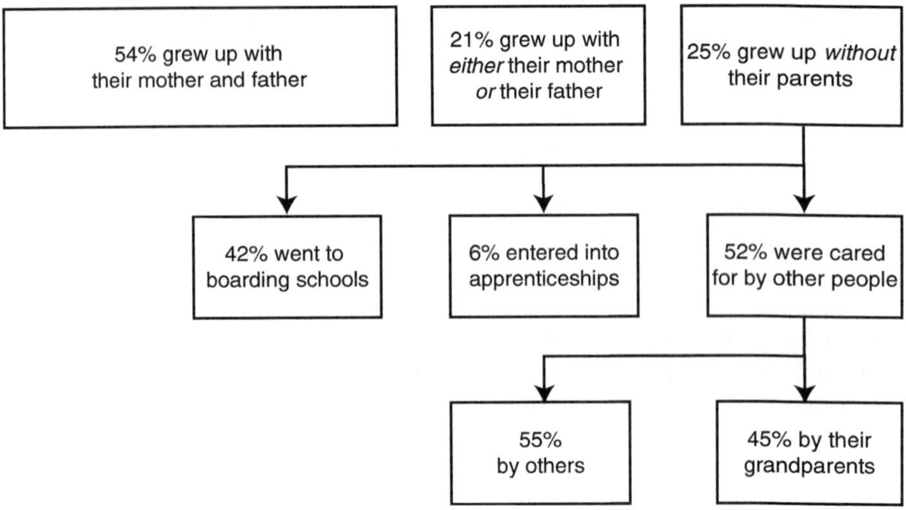

Fig. 7.1 Parental circumstances of respondents born between 1930 and 1950, up to age 14 (*Source*: *Biographies et entourage* survey, INED, 2001)

The identification of "resource persons" who took care of these children again shows the potential of blood relatives: almost half (44 %) of the children entrusted to third parties went to live (for at least a year) with their grandparents, who were thus the first point of call with respect to children's upbringing. This confirms the change described by Attias-Donfut and Segalen (1998, p. 233): "In short, there has been a shift from support for a limited number of grandchildren for a long time, in a parental mode, to broader support (in terms of the number of grandchildren) but of a lesser form and for limited periods of time" (Fig. 7.1).

7.5 Grandparents: From Role Model to Rejection

The analysis of the qualitative interviews in this second part of the chapter supports the idea of the essential role played by grandparents in respondents' childhood. The notion that they were somewhat forgotten or distant relatives is not borne out in the surveys considered here, contrary to the situation described by Attias-Donfut and Segalen (1998, p. 77): "barely 20 or 30 years ago, grandparents were not only ignored, but even elicited cautious reserve on the part of parents". Moreover, many respondents spent their youth in a family environment where grandparents had an important, even central, role.

Indeed, grandparents' roles, as we have seen, are far from restricted to those of the cake-baking grandparent, prominent in the vision of new grandparents. Grandparents may become role models or, on the contrary, elicit negative feelings of rejection. In both cases, they have profoundly influenced the trajectories of respondents, as we shall see in the following analyses.

7.5.1 Grandparents as an Example

When grandparents are seen as an example, their influence emerges clearly in the way respondents experience their own grandparenthood. Their approach is directly inspired by that of their own grandparents.

7.5.1.1 Cohabitation Between Generations in a Working-Class Context

Géraldine was born in 1936, married an electrician in the building industry, and has raised five children. In the questionnaire, she cited her grandmother as having played a parental role throughout her life. "During the war, she was a second mother." Indeed, the grandmother was an integral part of the family who followed her daughter from move to move.

> Oh yes, Grandmother was there all the time, Grandmother… was widowed very young and Mum had got married very young, and my grandmother always followed her, and us, my brother, my sister and me, it was my grandmother that raised us. And my grandmother always came with us.[6]

The grandmother's role is so important that, at key moments in Géraldine's life, it was to her that she turned.

> … oh, my grandmother, she was a wonderful person. Oh yes, my grandmother… I love my mum, you know, but it's Gran that takes precedence. When you had something to ask, you didn't go to Mum, you went to Gran. And when I found out I was pregnant, who came with me? Because I was really quite young, you know.

Throughout her life, Géraldine's grandmother was there for her granddaughter, in particular every winter, when she would spend several months with them, despite poor housing conditions.

> – Yes, she came to us for the winter. We couldn't be apart from her, she was her favourite daughter so… Yes, her favourite granddaughter.
> – So your grandmother who would come from Saint Malo.
> – From Saint Malo, yes. Stayed in the old house with us and, well, she liked it, she was contented, she was happy.

Now, after the death of her grandmother, it is her mother's turn to spend every winter staying with Géraldine's family.

[6] The following quotes are taken from the qualitative interviews.

I've taken up the baton, if you like. Mum had her mother to stay, and now I have my mother to stay over the winter… there you go. And so the cycle goes on.

So much so that Géraldine takes on the same role with one of her granddaughters by having her at home every day and taking her on holiday.

- Do you have your granddaughter every day?
- Oh, every day for the last eight years now. Except Saturdays and Sundays. . But otherwise… we take her on holiday with us, us… we take her everywhere, Justine, it's as if she was our own. Because we go on holiday in July, and then her parents go away in August. So she comes with us in July. And if we go to my daughter's in the Vendée, during the holidays, we take our granddaughter with us. I take here everywhere, Justine, well, it's as if she was me…, as if she was my youngest daughter. Yes, I often call her Valérie… I call her by the name of… because she resembles her aunt a lot, you know. Oh yes.

The relationship between grandmother and granddaughter is so close that a certain confusion of roles is once again evident, with a "blurring of generations". Géraldine considered her grandmother to be her mother in some ways, and now she likens her granddaughter to her daughter.

7.5.1.2 Family Holidays from Generation to Generation in an Affluent Middle-Class Context

Christine was born in 1936 in Marseille into a family of five children. Her father was an engineer, as was her grandfather, while her mother stayed at home. Christine has two key geographical attachments: Marseille, where she was born, and Grenoble, where her paternal grandmother bought a family holiday home, which she and her siblings have had to part with.

That's right, my other grandmother, my father's mother, she was from Grenoble, she'd bought a family home for us and her five children where, as used to be the custom in France, we would spend all our holidays, there was no question of going anywhere else or anything like that. We spent all our holidays with our… I don't know, I'd have to work it out, was it 14 or 17, we spent all our holidays with all our cousins… You could tell the whole history of our family by telling the story of that house.

For Christine, family necessarily means a large family centred on one or more houses. When she ended up living on her own with her youngest son in Amiens, she left there in order to join the rest of the family in Paris. But the Paris apartment was too small to accommodate her siblings and her children. So Christine, forced to sell the family home, sought to reproduce the model initiated by her grandmother by buying a second home in the Grenoble area, near to where her sister lives. The most important thing is to have a place where they can get together, in order to foster group cohesion and perpetuate the family spirit.

It's the pretty house in the village, where my elder sister lives and where I, that's very recent too, I've bought a house opposite… We're on the other side of the valley, we're 10 minutes away, I've bought a house, which we're in the process of doing up little by little and where my children come to visit. If you like, we're starting what we did in S. again, we're starting again on the other side of the valley, in V. So things carry on like that. And so the idea is that it's a house, the key's in a box by the front door and, if everything goes to plan, when it gradually starts to become inhabitable, well, the kids can go there, their friends can go there. My brothers and sisters can go there, all they need to do is put the key back in the same place and then I'll find everything as I left it, you know, but well it's really a wish I've had my whole life that's coming true, almost on a whim, you might say, and now I can't help thinking that… That's why I'm selling this flat. So it's really… Basically to return to the same kind of existence in a way, you know.

As Géraldine puts it, "and so the cycle goes on"; in Christine's words, "we're starting again". Each of them, in their own way, is reproducing the behaviours of their grandmothers, who made a strong impression on them. In the case of working-class Géraldine, this takes the form of intermittent cohabitation; in the case of Christine, from a more bourgeois background, it takes the form of the purchase of a family home in which to bring together children and grandchildren.

These examples represent extreme cases of transmission of grandparenthood that involve an "exact reproduction", whether by setting aside a room in the house for the grandmother and then the mother and the granddaughter, or by purchasing a family home. In most cases, the transmission of grandparenting does not occur in the same way, if only because several different lineages are involved. But as Attias-Donfut and Segalen write (1998, p. 216), "the memory of the grandparents is like a kind of founding memory that provides an identity-related resource to guide actions in the present". And, in reality, buying a second home is often linked to the desire to bring the family together, especially the grandchildren, in order to pass on a "family spirit" or to recreate one's family with children, stepchildren and grandchildren (Attias-Donfut et al. 2002; Clément and Bonvalet 2005).

7.5.2 Rejection

While in the vast majority of cases, grandparents leave respondents with fond memories and are often cited as attachment figures, we cannot ignore another, much less positive case. Again, we will only consider extreme examples. A distinction can be made between two types of case.

7.5.2.1 Respondents Who Distance Themselves from Their Grandparents and Their Families in General

This is the case for Anne, born in 1947 into a large family in northern France. From birth to the age of 5, she lived in her paternal grandmother's house; then, when her second sister was born, her parents went to stay with the maternal grandmother, where she remained until she was 8. She remembers that very intense family life, essentially focused on her mother's side of the family.

My mother's family, especially my grandmother, you know, we lived with them for a while, but afterwards (following a move) we would go on Thursdays, as we had the day off at the

> time. We would each go in turn. There were three of us and we'd each spend a Thursday there. We'd go on the Wednesday night… and we we'd go practically every Sunday. Christmas was a big event, when everyone was there. Family life was very intense.

Anne's narrative begins like those of many respondents, which evoke such family gatherings with warmth. But very quickly the tone changes and the family is described as suffocating – a fact that would ultimately lead her to break away from her family, which was organized into "clans".

> My mother's family took up an enormous amount of space in our lives, which incidentally led to a lot of rebellion inside me because I hate clan mentalities. So in the end I left for Paris and it's true that I was happy at that time but there comes a point where I just can't be doing with clans…

Carole has similar memories, namely of her maternal grandmother being very much present – too present, even. Cohabitation and geographic proximity between parents and grandparents made family life suffocating for her too.

- Oh, my grandmother in any case was always there, ever-present… that was terrible, really, because it was a constant reminder that she wanted to be taken care of by her daughter. Well, there was a funny story, because my grandmother was widowed during the First World War and she only had my mother. It's a very odd story and then, goodness me, my mother, over time she's become a friend, they had a funny relationship, and also a relationship of dependency that was really very strong, I'd say unhealthy, that's for sure… What happened in fact was that, well, it's true that as soon as I got my Solex [a kind of moped], the atmosphere at home, at my parents' at least at that time, it was really, oh, truly awful for me… yes and so the Solex was just fabulous because it was an instrument of freedom, of movement… and also a way to get out of this house where I felt so awful.
- And was it more your mother or your father?
- Oh no, it was the atmosphere in general, you know, maintained I would say by my ever-present grandmother who, even from a distance, controlled my mother.

From this point on, Carole could only think about escaping from the family home. A friend and the moped would help her achieve this, but she nevertheless has negative memories of her adolescence, which she describes as difficult.

7.5.2.2 Rejection of Respondents by Their Grandparents

Grandchildren who have suffered from overbearing family relationships may reject their families and their grandparents, but the rejection can also work in the opposite direction. Grandparents may reject their grandchildren after a souring of their relationship with their adult children. This is often the case with "unsuitable marriages" (e.g. marrying beneath one's social class), shotgun weddings in particular.

- I saw my grandfather more often than my grandmother and my grandmother was a nasty lady.
- You saw your grandfather more often?
- He would often pop in. He would pop in. He would often come to the house.
- But not so much your grandmother?
- Absolutely not, no.
- Why not?

- Why not? Because, because... basically... we were the black sheep of the family, you know. Which is to say that there was... my parents got married because my mother was pregnant. And you know, at the time, that really wasn't great, I was born in'44... Yes, that's right, two months, and my paternal grandmother was very angry about it, and in any case believed that my mother had in some way cheated on my father, which is to say that I wasn't... so there was this other thing too, I was the bastard, you know. There you go. But for my brothers, my brothers were OK, you know, because they were born legitimately I suppose you could say. There you go. But not me, so the less everyone saw of me, the happier they were, you know!
- So you felt this disapproval from your grandmother?
- Oh, it wasn't that I felt it, it was that she called me "the bastard".
- Ah.
- Yes. And when you're little, you don't always understand what words mean, so I understood a bit later, when I was 7 or 8, you know, so I tried to understand... I mean understand why, you know. My mother explained to me that she got married when she was pregnant, so there you go. So I understood. And so afterwards, the less I saw of her, the happier I was too, you know.

Laure talks about "unjustified violence towards her" – violence that was exacerbated by the fact that, as the daughter of a manual worker, she found herself shunned by the pupils at the high school in the neighbouring town, attended by the children of farmers and traders. "The feeling of injustice is something I experienced very early on." Laure studied to become a social worker, but failed the exams. She later worked in the social sector and return to higher education.

> And I got my DEA [master's degree]. So I was quite proud of myself, at age 47! You know. And then... well I got so much satisfaction that I told myself: right, in a way I've got my revenge, I've got one over on life. I'm sorry, that could come across as being a bit strong but...

At 50, Laure is involved in the French communist party and is a local councillor in a municipality in the Paris suburbs – but, despite all this, she remains, in her words, "the black sheep of the family: an intellectual in a family of manual workers stands out like a sore thumb." She is divorced and has a daughter, who is also in higher education and with whom she is very close.

In Laure's case, the feeling of injustice she harbours originated in her grandmother's rejection of her during childhood, and then persisted at school and in her professional and political life. It is therefore very much a question of this "kind of founding memory that provides an identity-related resource to guide actions in the present" (Attias-Donfut and Segalen 1998, p. 216), but with a pattern that radically differs from those of Christine and Géraldine.

7.6 Conclusion

While grandparents have long been forgotten by researchers in France, the respondents in the *Biographies et entourage* survey attest to the influence of their grandparents, whose roles varied significantly, ranging from taking care of everything (including acting as foster parents), living in multi-generational household and "close protection", on the one hand, to family relationships that might be more distant, or even in a state of breakdown, on the other. The modernity of these grandparents does not lie in a new "cake-baking" role, as has been suggested by certain American and French researchers. Rather, these grandparents represent continuity, not modernity.

Most surprisingly, the baby-boom generations continue to take on the role of grandparent in the same way as their parents and grandparents did before them. By passing on the family memory in this manner, they ensure the continued existence of a bridge between generations, and meet the "need for roots and origins" (Gourdon 2001) of the youngest family members while also respecting their desire for independence. With the rise of individualism, these generations might have been expected to favour circles of professional contacts and friends, and invest less energy in the family realm. Their modernity lies in the fact that they are able to do both.

References

Attias-Donfut, C., & Segalen, M. (1998). *Grands-parents : la famille à travers les générations*. Paris: Éditions Odile Jacob.
Attias-Donfut, C., Segalen, M., & Lapierre, N. (2002). *Le nouvel esprit de famille*. Paris: Éditions Odile Jacob.
Bois, J.-P. (1991). L'art d'être grand-mère, au XVIIe-XIXe siècle. *Annales de démographie historique*, 7–19.
Bonvalet, C., & Ogg, J. (2007). *Measuring family support in Europe*. London: Southern Universities Press.
Burguière, A., Klapisch-Zuber, C., Segalen, M., & Zonabend, F. (Eds.). (1986). *Histoire de la famille, I. Mondes lointains, mondes anciens, II. Le choc des modernités*. Paris: Armand Colin.
Cichelli-Pugeault, O., & Cicchelli, V. (1998). *Les théories sociologiques de la famille*. Paris: La Découverte, coll. "Repères".
Clément, C., & Bonvalet, C. (2005). Familles recomposées et ancrage résidentiel : le rôle de la résidence secondaire. *Espaces et sociétés*, numéro 120–121, pp. 79–97.
Collectif. (1975). *Finie la famille ? Traditions et nouveaux rôles*. Paris: Autrement.
Comte, A. (1995 [1839]). *Cours de philosophie positive*. Paris: Flammarion.
Cooper, D. (1972). *Mort de la famille*. Paris: Seuil.
de Singly, F. (1991). *La famille : état des savoirs*. Paris: La Découverte.
de Singly, F. (1993a). Comment définir la famille contemporaine? *Études statistiques, 4*, 31–39.
de Singly, F. (1993b). *Sociologie de la famille contemporaine*. Paris: Nathan.
de Tocqueville, A. (1835). *De la démocratie en Amérique*. Paris: Flammarion.
Durkheim, E. (1892). La famille conjugale. In E. Durkheim (Ed.), *1975, Le sens commun. Textes III : fonctions sociales et institutions*. Paris: Éditions de Minuit.
Durkheim, E. (1975). *Le sens commun. Textes III : fonctions sociales et institutions*. Paris: Éditions de Minuit.
Foisil, M. (1991). Grands-pères de jadis XVIIe-XIXe siècles. Quelques modèles. *Annales de démographie historique*, 51–63.
Gokalp, C. (1978). Le réseau familial. *Population, 33*(6), 1077–1094.
Gourdon, V. (2001). *Histoire des grands-parents*. Paris: Perrin.

Le Bras, H. (1973). Parents, grands-parents, bisaïeux. *Population, 28*(1), 9–38.
Lelièvre, E., & Vivier, G. (2001). Evaluation d'une collecte à la croisée du quantitatif et du qualitatif, l'enquête *Biographies et entourage. Population, 56*(6), 1043–1074.
Lelièvre, E., Vivier, G., & Tichit, C. (2008). Between socially-instituted parental relationships and elective ones: A retrospective analysis of parent figures in France from 1930 to 1965. *Population, English Edition, 63*(2), 209–238.
Parsons, T. (1943). The kinship system of the contemporary United States. *American Anthropologist, 45* pp. 22–38.
Pitrou, A. (1978). *Vivre sans famille*. Toulouse: Privat.
Roussel, L. (1976). La famille après le mariage des enfants : les relations entre générations. *Population, 31*(6), 1195–1206.
Stone, L. (1977). *The family, sex and marriage in England. 1500–1800*. New York: Harper & Row.
Théry, I. (Ed.). (1995). *Recomposer une famille, des rôles et des sentiments*. Paris: Éditions Textuel.
Théry, I. (1998). *Couple, filiation et parenté aujourd'hui. Le droit face aux mutations de la famille et de la vie privée*. Paris: Éditions Odile Jacob.
Weber, F. (2002). Pour penser la parenté contemporaine. In D. Debordeaux & R. Strobel (Eds.), *Les Solidarités familiales en questions : entraide et transmission* (Vol. 34, pp. 73–106). Paris: Maison des Sciences de l'Homme, coll. "Droit et société".
Young, M., & Willmott, R. (1957). *Family and kinship in East London*. London: Routledge and Kegan Paul.

Chapter 8
Stepfamilies and Residential Rootedness

Céline Clément and Catherine Bonvalet

Since the 1970s, many significant changes in family and conjugal life have been observed. In particular, there has been a rapid increase in the number of divorces, and a trend towards "new" family configurations, such as single-parent households and stepfamilies, together with a tendency for individuals to experience a succession of "family sequences" throughout their lives, challenging the image of a uniform, stable and sustainable family model, and thus also the notion of the family within the restricted context of the household. While stepfamilies have always existed, as various historical studies show (Burguière 1993; Flandrin 1984), the conditions governing their formation have changed: today, they are more often associated with divorce than with the death of a parent, and in these cases children often maintain links with both parents. As stepfamilies resulting from divorce have become more common, new questions have arisen, in particular regarding the role of the father, the mother, the stepfather and the stepmother – who have to take on "new" functions (Théry 1987, 1996; Le Gall 1996; Le Gall and Martin 1993; Blöss 1996, 1997; Cadolle 2000; Martial 2003) – but also with regard to the very definition of the family, which now "extends beyond the four walls of the home". Sociologists and demographers have had to re-examine the concept of the family by looking past the strict confines of the household and therefore also of co-residence (Desplanques 1994; Bonvalet and Lelièvre 1995; Bonvalet 1997; de Singly 1997). With this in

Research supported by PUCA (Plan Urbanisme Construction Architecture) as part of the "Habitat et vie urbaine" (Housing and Urban Life) programme. This article was initially published in the journal *Espaces et Sociétés* under the title "La famille dans tous ses espaces", 2005, 120 (1–2), pp. 79–97.

C. Clément
Centre de recherches sociologiques et politiques de Paris (Cresppa-GTM), Université Paris Ouest Nanterre La Défense, Nanterre, France

C. Bonvalet (✉)
Institut national d'études démographiques (INED), Paris, France
e-mail: bonvalet@ined.fr

C. Bonvalet, É. Lelièvre (eds.), *Family Beyond Household and Kin*,
INED Population Studies 6, DOI 10.1007/978-3-319-24684-0_8

mind, the definition of the family, which traditionally includes only related individuals who live in the same dwelling, would no longer seem to be relevant: children from stepfamilies have seen their "territory" increase in size, typically by a factor of two or more. In addition to the limitations associated with the "classic" definition of the family, research on stepfamilies has also highlighted the limits of an excessively static vision of the realities of many families, and has underlined the importance of including a temporal dimension in the analysis – for example, by seeking to describe the different sequences of family life and the way in which these follow on from one another. As the family structures observed at any given moment are the result of a process, only longitudinal analyses make it possible to assess the "imprint of life trajectories" (Blöss 1996). As a result, sociologists and demographers eventually proposed that the statistical concept of the family be broadened, beyond the notion of co-residence, and extended to the entire family network resulting from parents' conjugal trajectories. Stepfamilies are today defined as family "constellations" determined by children's movements between paternal and maternal households, where the dimensions of space and time appear to be of fundamental importance (Théry; Blöss; Cadolle; Le Gall and Martin; Martial – op. cit.).

Nevertheless, these studies are still essentially focused on the primary residence of the parents or step-parents – a level of analysis that is simply insufficient. As several studies on the family and housing have underlined, it is necessary to move away from the vision of a single family dwelling and instead take account of multiple places of residence over long periods in people's lives (Bonnin and de Villanova 1999). Isabelle Bertaux-Wiame (1995), for example, highlighted the need to take the wider family context into consideration. A phenomenon of multiple residence is at play here, in all social categories, with "secondary" residences "occupying an important place [in family life], in material, social and symbolic terms". The inhabited space is therefore not restricted to the primary residence and "can take the form of a residential archipelago" (Bonnin and de Villanova, op. cit.). Furthermore, while studies have shown how a second residence can give structure to a family identity, the true extent of this symbolic role for stepfamilies needs to be verified. To this end, the purchase of a second home or evidence of significant time spent in a place of "rootedness" (e.g. the primary residence of grandparents or an aunt, or a holiday home) can also be indicators of families that function in this kind of way, seeking to establish, build and maintain links between children and stepchildren, between siblings, half-siblings and stepsiblings, as well as between grandchildren. It is for this reason that notions of living spaces (Courgeau 1975; Frémont et al. 1984) and residential systems (Pinson 1988; Barbary and Dureau 1993), alongside phenomena of multiple residence with movements and links between each dwelling, are proposed in this article. These concepts – which extend beyond the prism of the usual place of residence and include all places frequented – therefore allow us to follow, in time and space, not just one location but several, which may change over the course of individuals' trajectories. Consequently, while co-residence and the "shared experiences of childhood" stand out as the bedrock of relationships between parents, children, step-parents, stepchildren – and above all between siblings, half-siblings and stepsiblings (Martial 2003; Poittevin 2003) – we shall focus here on the different places, past and present, frequented by the members of a stepfamily, and the values that are attached to these places via the family relationships associated with them.

8.1 The Research Project

8.1.1 The Biographies et entourage *Survey*

This research project takes the form of a qualitative survey of individuals with stepfamilies. The starting point for the interviews was the questionnaire-based *Biographies et entourage* survey conducted by INED. This survey, which collected data relating to the occupational, residential and family histories of its respondents, concerned individuals from birth cohorts born between 1930 and 1950.[1] It explores the entourage of these respondents: members of their descent group (father, mother, children, grandchildren), collateral relatives (siblings, half-siblings, stepsiblings) and affines (life partners, parents and children thereof), as well as any individuals who have lived with the respondent for at least a year and any other individuals cited by the respondent as having played a key role – positive or negative – in his or her life. For this last group, only family events and occupational histories were recorded. The questionnaire asks for details of three generations, with respondents forming the pivotal generation. In addition to this description of the respondent's entourage, the survey collected details of every family and occupational event known to the respondent, and all dwellings occupied by the respondent since birth. Of the 2,830 individuals surveyed, 21 % had been in more than one consensual union. If we consider those respondents who have children and/or stepchildren (i.e. children of their life partner) resulting from a previous union, as well as those respondents with children born outside a consensual union, we arrive at a figure of 628 individuals with stepfamilies – either at the time of the survey or at some other point in the course of their family trajectory – or 22 % of all respondents. However, there are several ways in which respondents may be deemed to belong to a stepfamily[2]: first, a respondent with children from a previous union (or born outside a consensual union) may form a union with a partner who has never been in a union before (38 %); second, a respondent who has never been in a relationship before may form a union with someone who has children from a previous union (29 %); and third, both partners may have children from previous unions (33 %).

[1] Each questionnaire systematically collected detailed descriptions relating to a varied circle of people and places, as well as the family, occupational and residential trajectories of the respondent and his or her parents and life partners – amounting to some 11,000–12,000 interconnected life event histories.

[2] In this research, the standpoint adopted is that of respondents who are parents. For example, a single divorced woman who has two children does not belong to a stepfamily, even if the father of her children is in a union with someone else (however, her children *do* belong to a stepfamily).

8.1.2 The Interviews

In this chapter, the sample population is limited to respondents born between 1940 and 1950, who are in the "intermediate occupations" category and who have at some point had a stepfamily.[3] It might be presumed that these middle-class stepfamilies tended to function more on the basis of a substitution model – characterized by the formation of a new family that supplants the previous one – than today's stepfamilies, which typically tend to function on the basis of a continuity model, where relations of some sort are maintained within the parental couple (Théry 1987; Le Gall and Martin 1993). Nevertheless, analysis of these cohorts will enable us to take the long-term situation into consideration and observe changes in the way these families function between the separation of the parental couple and the entry into adulthood of the children and stepchildren. It will then be possible to identify the different processes involved in the formation of a stepfamily over time, with respect to housing and spatial considerations, insofar as these processes change and adapt according to the context. Note that it was not always easy to define someone as having formed a stepfamily, as certain family configurations could be somewhat disorganized or variable in nature (Le Gall and Martin 1988a). We focused first on individuals who had been through a divorce or separation, excluding those whose partners had died. Several questions then enabled us to identify those respondents who had since formed a new union, as well as those who had been in a "part-time" union and those who had experienced a second break-up. Next, the questionnaire provided information about the children: their family events, their place of residence, and also the frequency of contact between respondents and their children. We should point out at this juncture that some male respondents from these cohorts indicated that they no longer had any contact with their children from a previous union. In some cases, they specified that this had been the case since the divorce, while in other cases we had no way of knowing whether contact had ended more recently – in particular at the time of the survey. These individuals were excluded, even in cases where they had since entered into a new union and now had stepchildren, as their situations tended to reflect a rationale of substitution, "a sort of social widowerhood" typical of first divorces (Théry 1991). We nonetheless decided to interview female respondents who reported that they no longer had any contact with their ex-partner and that this ex-partner had since "acquired a stepfamily". We worked on the initial assumption that breaking off relations with the former partner did not automatically lead to a lack of contact between the non-custodial parent and his or her children. Indeed, regarding contact between ex-partners and their children, while several questionnaires recorded that contact had ended between the two parents now separated, subsequent interviews showed that the children had nevertheless maintained relations with their father and/or other members of the paternal

[3] The "intermediate occupations" category was selected because, even in cases where housing conditions are limited by budgetary and spatial constraints, these individuals nevertheless have some room for manoeuvre in their residential choices and geographical attachments.

family. This discrepancy can be explained in large part by the wording of the question which is put to one of the parents about contacts with their ex-partner (co-parent of the children): "Currently (or before his/her death), how often did you have contact with one another?" We can assume that ex-partners who maintained contact purely for practical reasons and for important decisions relating to their children break off all relations once the children enter adulthood (Le Gall and Martin 1988b).

Finally, given the limited number of interviews, the survey presented here cannot be considered as representative, and no generalizations can be made based on these observations. It does, however, provide an opportunity to examine stepfamilies at a different scale – that of living spaces – and to explore new methodological avenues. Accordingly, we collected histories and narratives from men and women relating to their residential trajectories, where the common factor was the experience of forming a stepfamily. Nine women born between 1941 and 1950 and six men born between 1941 and 1948 were interviewed. These semi-structured interviews lasted 2 h on average.

8.2 Moving Between Spaces: The Question of Custody

Before addressing the question of places frequented, we ought first to take a closer look at the relations between ex-partners, particularly in terms of custody arrangements following a divorce. In the cohorts studied (1940–1950), alternating custody was rare.[4] We might therefore expect the practice of alternating residence to have been non-existent, with primary custody granted to mothers – a choice made as much by fathers as by mothers, although it would perhaps be more accurate to talk about a lack of choice, as this option seemed to "go without saying" in view of the social representations of the period. In the interviews, some women mentioned sporadic contact between their children and their father. In several cases, stepmothers appeared to be the "cause" of the breakdown of the relationship between father and children, or of a reduced frequency of contact at the very least. Nonetheless, their testimonies indicate that they would like their children to pursue this contact. In some cases, legal action was taken. But, more generally, when respondents were asked about the custody of their children, they saw it as perfectly natural for the mother to have primary custody, with the father seeing his children during school

[4] Prior to 1975, when divorce by mutual consent was made legal in France, one parent was typically granted sole custody of any children, to the exclusion of the other, with the decision made in reference to matrimonial fault. After this date, the practice of alternating custody (today called alternating residence in France) became more widespread, but only marginally so. It was prohibited by a judgement of the French Court of Cassation on 2 May 1984. The "Malhuret law" of 22 July 1987 then legalized the principle of joint exercise of parental authority by both divorced parents, albeit with one residence designated as the child's habitual residence. In 1993, this measure was extended to cohabiting parents. The French law of 4 March 2002 formalized alternating residence.

holidays and at weekends. This notwithstanding, five interviews reveal cases where custody was granted to the father. These were very often the result of "atypical" situations. Françoise, for example, did not obtain custody of her second daughter, born during a second union (she had a first daughter from a previous union). When she divorced a second time in 1985, her husband obtained custody of their daughter and kept the house, which was in his name. This was part of a "deal" arranged by him. However, contrary to the stated conditions of this deal, once Françoise became more stable psychologically, financially and residentially, she did not regain custody of her second daughter, underlining the complexity of the legal system. She saw her only at weekends and during school holidays. Her first daughter on the other hand, had not wished to live with either her ex-stepfather or her mother, preferring instead to live with her maternal aunt. The interviews also reveal men's situations, such as that of Alain, who requested custody of his son from a second union, in an arrangement drawn up with his ex-partner (they were not married) who was now living in a union with another woman; he wished to offer his son a different image of the parental couple while enabling mother and son to maintain their relationship. In some cases, siblings do not share the same primary residence; one or more may live with their mother and the other(s) with their father. Jacques, for example, obtained primary custody of his son, while his daughters remained with their mother. However, looking beyond the custody arrangements laid down by the law, we observe a great deal of flexibility and movement, initiated by the children, particularly when they are teenagers and/or when parents have to deal with other problems (financial, health-related, etc.). The legal decision does not, therefore, always reflect what happens in practice. For instance, one of Jacques' daughters decided to move in with him in her teenage years when she was in conflict with her mother. Similarly, when Emmanuelle divorced in 1986, she obtained primary custody of her two daughters. Nevertheless, her daughters, and also her stepdaughters, often moved back and forth between her home and her ex-husband's home throughout their teenage years. This is a prime example of how children sometimes move between their parents' residences, for varying periods of time and with varying degrees of permanence. The same phenomenon is illustrated by a previous study concerning the children of divorced parents, which revealed that children's patterns of movement between different parental homes changed as they got older and as parent-child relationships evolved (Clément 2002, 2009). Parents may therefore make extralegal arrangements "in the child's interest" – a fact that may go unnoticed in a quantitative study, as highlighted by Sylvie Cadolle (2003).

8.3 Relations and Encounters Between Ex-Partners

While the interviews did not suggest that the substitution model (Théry 1996) was dominant (none of the children of those interviewed had broken off contact with their non-custodial parent), an "intermediate model" can be defined, where children and non-custodial parents keep in touch and maintain a relationship, as in the continuity model, but where ex-partners avoid meeting and essentially communicate through the children. This model is linked to the age of the children when their parents separate: typically, they are teenagers and so are more able to manage their relationships with their parents and their movements between different residences, as underlined by Didier Le Gall and Claude Martin (1988a): adolescence seems to lead to a greater recognition of each household (that of the custodial parent and that of the non-custodial parent) as separate entities. There is a clear separation between the conjugal couple on the one hand and the parental couple on the other, but bonds of filiation are maintained, with the child forming the link between the two. Sometimes, parents try not to meet at all, even when dropping off or picking up their children from one another's home. This was the case, for example, for Françoise, who waited in the car when picking up her two daughters from their father's home, and for Emmanuelle, who never met her ex-partner, despite living in the same locality as him, and whose daughters were old enough to make their own way between their respective homes.

Relations between ex-partners that extend beyond questions such as education and visiting schedules are very rare. As pointed out by Jacques – who obtained primary custody of his son at the time of the divorce and, later on, of one of his daughters when she was 15 – arrangements were made to ensure that the siblings met up every weekend and during school holidays. Relations remained "tense", however, and focused exclusively on their children. Children's weddings and grandchildren's christenings are therefore occasions when everyone can "get together", in an atmosphere which, while not exactly warm, nevertheless remains "courteous". And ultimately, even in cases where parents do not meet, they receive news of one another via their children. Building friendly relations is clearly difficult, however. For the interviewees, it is important for each person – parents and step-parents alike – to know their place and to not compete with parental figures. Even in cases where respondents do not indicate a breakdown in relations, this does not mean they wish to meet with their ex-partner. Where meetings do take place, they rarely occur in either of the ex-partners' homes, which are considered private, intimate spaces. Lastly, a few respondents have not only maintained a relationship as parents, but also established relations of friendship and sometimes even support. However, these situations are generally the exception rather than the rule. This is the case for Évelyne, for example, who maintains numerous links with her partner's ex-stepfamily. Nevertheless, this type of relationship may be facilitated by Évelyne's lack of family history, as she has never had children herself (Blöss 1996, 1997; Cadolle 2000).

8.4 Paternal Grandparents: A Stable and Lasting Link

Lack of contact between ex-partners does not always lead to a breakdown of ties with their ex-families-in-law. While most respondents no longer maintain such ties, others pursue them, in particular with their ex-parents-in-law. This is the case for

Isabelle, for example. Throughout her marriage, she regularly went to her ex-parents-in-law's house, in provincial France, with her children. Although now divorced from their son, she has not cut off ties with them. They often invite her to stay with them, along with her children. However, Isabelle now wants to "loosen" these ties, as their house is "the [children's] father's house" and to "break away" from this aspect of her personal life in order to mark a clear separation: "I no longer feel at home there," she says, clearly placing this family home in the context of a descent group to which she no longer belongs. Nevertheless, she continues to visit her ex-parents-in-law once or twice a year.

More surprising is the case of Daniel, the father of three daughters from two marriages, and the stepfather of two children from a third union. Although originally from Marseille, which is home to his family and his ex-partners, he currently lives in Saint-Quentin-en-Yvelines (a new town in the south-western outer suburbs of Paris), with his third wife. He first married at age 18, and had a daughter, but divorced very soon after. He had no further contact with his first wife, or indeed with his daughter. A year after his divorce, aged 21, he married again and had two more daughters. Two years later, he divorced a second time and moved to Bourg-la-Reine (in the southern inner suburbs of Paris), where he moved in with his third partner who already had two children. He nonetheless remained in contact with his second wife and their two daughters in Marseille. Figure 8.1 shows the role played by Marseille in Daniel's life.[5] We can see that meetings with his daughters take place at the homes of either his mother or his sister, both of whom live in Marseille, as do his daughters and ex-partners. Remarkably, his mother has always kept in touch with his first daughter:

[5] The diagrams in this chapter were created using the Réseau-lu® software designed by André Mogoutov. They are life-event diagrams that seek to highlight the internal organization of trajectories described in terms of a succession of states and events linked to family-related factors (births, union formations, weddings, cohabitation with children and partners) or residential factors (migration, different places of residence, places frequented, secondary residences, etc.). The software first identifies the states for a given year and the events that occurred in the course of that year. For example, Fig. 8.1 shows, in the lower right-hand corner, the move to Bourg-la-Reine, the formation of the third union, and cohabitation with the new partner's children. At this stage in the process, temporal aspects are considered implicitly: the number of links observed depends on the duration of a given state. The longer the duration of a state, the greater the probability that this state is contemporaneous with other states of the trajectory. For each state or event, the software calculates a centrality index (the number of links for the state or event divided by the total number of possible links). All the states/events are then ordered according to their centrality index and the diagram is constructed using an iterative process that positions states and events starting with the most linked and ending with the most isolated; this means that the absence of links between states and events already positioned in the diagram leads to a distancing of non-contemporaneous states (e.g. the birth of the first daughter has no link with the move to Bourg-la-Reine, and so the two points are positioned some distance apart). Those elements that are linked to several different stages of marital life, such as Marseille and the parents, are placed in the centre of the diagram. In this case, Marseille is linked to the first two unions, as they took place there, but also has a link with the third union, in that Daniel returns to the city regularly to see his mother and his daughters. The ellipses corresponding to each of the three conjugal periods were added in order to facilitate the interpretation of the diagram.

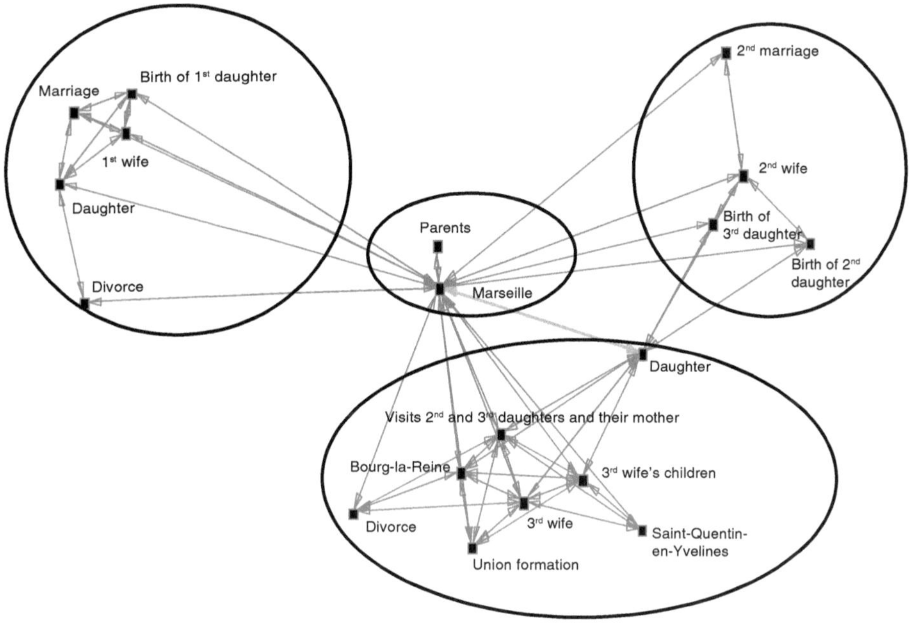

Fig. 8.1 Daniel's family and residential trajectories

So I got married at 18, at 20 I was divorced, I had a daughter, who's now about 40, she must be 40, and who stayed with her mother, and who I lost… Her mother didn't want her to see me… but all that, it's not really a big deal… and besides, I'm back in touch with her again now, and she's an extraordinary girl.

- And how old was she when you got back in touch with her?
- Oh, well, I hadn't [completely] lost contact with her, she still [saw] my mother, her grandmother, but not me. And then at my mother's 80th birthday, three years ago now, she was there. She's extraordinary but, you know, I have two other daughters who are also extraordinary. I only have daughters. So my second wife… well, there was a first wife with whom I had a daughter, we separated, well, I say separated… we went through a bitter divorce! I must have been 20, it was 40 years ago, very bitter! Ridiculous really! But anyway… because me, when I'm in love, I get married. So I met a girl when I was 21, and I had to marry her, same thing, I had two kids with her, two daughters who I adore.

(Daniel, born in 1944, sales technician)

His three daughters from his two unions know each other: only Daniel did not see his first daughter. Marseille is the common factor that unites the whole family, and indeed it is at Daniel's mother's home that the children meet up, together with Daniel's stepchildren and current partner.

- And in Marseille, you would see them at your mother's home?
- At my mother's, yes. At my mother's and at my sister's. Not at their mother's, you know, because, well, I had the good grace not to go round there. No but I would go down to Marseille every three months, and I would take them for the day, for two days, so at my mother's, yes. Yes, it was at my mother's.

- So they were still in contact with their grandmother?
- Oh yes, and they still are today. It's her that, well, not her, as my sister looks after my mother, but they see my mother once a week now, they've got children of their own. No, no, that's all gone very, very well. I tell you, considering the wife I had, their grandmother was... but even my first, my first wife, blimey! She never stopped my first daughter from seeing her grandmother, whom she saw a lot at the start when she was young, a bit less later on, but she never lost contact with my mother. No... so there you go, and that took place at my mother's, yes, because... yes, that's right... or at my sister's. My sister has a nice house near Marseille and so when I was at my sister's, I would pick up my daughters from my wife, you know, we'd go down there, even with my wife's children, we'd all turn up there, so they know each other well.

The paternal grandmother is the bedrock of the family relationships here, and it is through her and her home that the parental link is maintained. This confirms the observations made by Sylvie Cadolle (2003) concerning mutual support in stepfamily systems and the role of the paternal grandmother, sometimes maintained via the mother.

8.5 Places Frequented

As Aude Poittevin (2003) points out in her study of stepsiblings, "in this type of sibling configuration, co-residence is central as it becomes the factor that all the children have in common. Their surnames are different and don't reflect any shared family identity. What unites them is no longer their surname but their address." Agnès Martial (2003) also showed that the "shared experiences of childhood" appeared to be more important than biological characteristics such as whether they shared the same womb or the same blood. She also specified the foundational characteristics of the common household. A number of surveys underline how difficult it can be to "bring the children together": the absence of shared "history", "culture" or "values", or even of "family traditions", is often evoked. Indeed, it is for one such reason that Jeannette preferred to wait until her children had moved out before setting up home with her partner.

> But each of us did our own thing. We finished the job before moving in together. I had three, he had one. So there was no question of the children... I mean, divorces are hard enough as it is... if you force the children to mix together as well, it's not always... it's not always a success either. And in order to ensure a successful outcome, and today we realize that this is what it takes, we had to perhaps sacrifice 10 years, just over 10 years, more than that even, as we waited until the children had all finished their education, so bearing in mind they finished at 25, that must make it 15 years that we lived apart, each of us in our own home like that, we each raised our own children and today, well, now we both have grandchildren, and we've mixed everyone together and the children get on very, very well, there's no hatred, no ill feeling, everyone... so we've been rewarded for our efforts on that score.
> (Jeannette, born in 1950, accountant)

In this example, if we consider the periods when the children and stepchildren were young, we might suppose that these children spent little time together, as

Jeannette and her partner decided to move in together only much later on: their children had no experience of co-residence. And yet, by approaching the analysis from a different angle and including a temporal dimension in addition to the different places frequented outside the paternal and maternal residences, the role of holiday homes and secondary residences in creating and developing family ties between the different family members becomes clear. In this context, secondary residences or holiday homes can represent a means of creating "shared experiences". If we return to the example of Jeannette, we observe the importance of her partner's house in Brittany, where their grandchildren – who have brought the family together – come to stay. Although their respective children never spent time under the same roof during their childhood and teenage years, their "team of seven grandchildren" – their "troop" – comes together in this secondary residence. Furthermore, the couple are planning to move to Brittany permanently when Jeannette retires. If we turn to Alain and his wife, they emphasize the idea of "shared moments" experienced by their respective children from different unions. With this in mind, they have sought to create enjoyable moments together as a stepfamily in familiar "reference locations": every year, they go to the same place on holiday, in Normandy, in order to give their children "fixed bearings". The experience of "fragmented time" between siblings and half-siblings led Jacques to create other forms of sociability in different places: his workplace, for example, but also his secondary residence and his motor home.

8.6 The Role of Secondary Residences

Stepfamilies have to address the question of the home – or homes – because the "territories" in which children live are multiplied by a factor of two or more. As Didier Le Gall and Claude Martin point out (1991), "the question of housing and the home is integral to the process of stepfamily formation [...]." By investigating stepfamilies' use of domestic space, the authors showed just how much an analysis of the home – and more specifically who lives where, how the home is organized and how the domestic space is shared – can tell us about the way these families function. From this, they identified a number of rationales of stepfamily formation and various residential trajectories where the home "[...] contributes to the processes of regulation, and hence of cohesion, of the new family." Bearing this in mind, it might be useful to explore the of role secondary residences in the lives of stepfamilies.

The stepfamilies interviewed in the *Biographies et entourage* survey were not more likely to possess a secondary residence than other families: some 40 % of married couples had a second home, compared with 34 % of current stepfamilies (at the time of the survey) and 21 % of respondents who had formed a stepfamily at some point in their family trajectory.

Let us consider the examples of Isabelle, Christophe and Hélène, who all purchased secondary residences at some point during the formation of their respective stepfamilies, and whose unions were all still intact at the time of the survey.

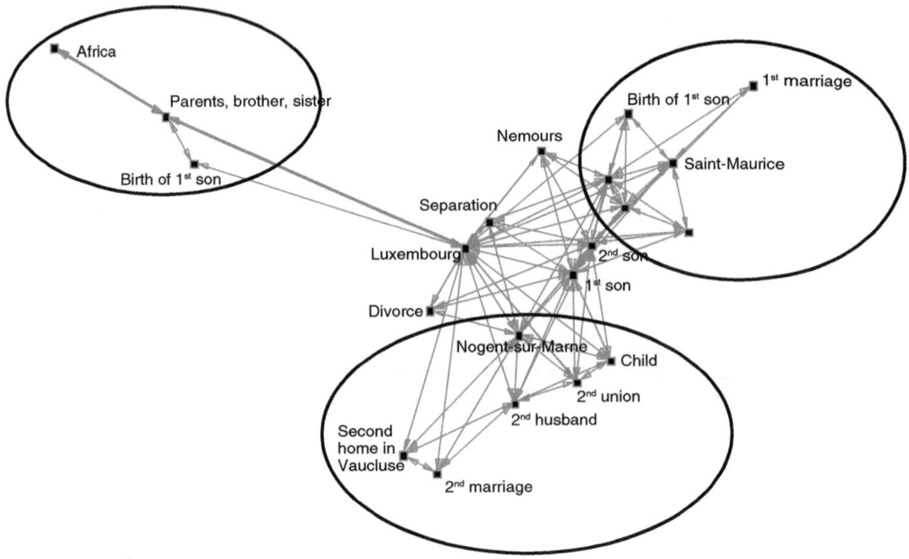

Fig. 8.2 Isabelle's family and residential trajectories

The cases of Isabelle (Fig. 8.2) and Christophe have a number of similarities: specifically, both purchased a secondary residence with their respective current partners.

Isabelle divorced in 1982. She received custody of her children and kept the apartment that she had bought in Nogent-sur-Marne (in the eastern inner suburbs of Paris). When she met her current partner in 1987, they agreed to continue living in their respective apartments. They then set up a system for spending time at each other's homes: Isabelle's partner would typically come to Nogent-sur-Marne, as her children were not there during the week. In 1990, her partner, a widower, and his younger son moved in with Isabelle. In 1993, the couple bought a secondary residence in the Vaucluse *département* in Provence. Here, it is interesting to note the role played by this house, in terms of residential, conjugal and family trajectories: the construction and decoration of the house is portrayed as a project for the couple – a "joint project" that was later formalized by holding their wedding there.

> [...] so as the house was built, yes, we fancied getting married there. In a way it tied up something that we'd done together.
>
> – Did it represent a joint project?
> – Yes. And I'm not saying that a house is like a baby, it isn't... But I think it's quite nice when you get remarried like that later in life, to have accomplished something together. There's something that... it's something that brings our two families together, this house, it's something we've done together. And I think it has clearly strengthened quite a few things. This joint project, which wasn't that easy to achieve, as we had to discuss things, make compromises, on both sides, such as who wants a bedroom here, who wants one there. So it's quite nice, I think, I think it's an opportunity, as we're not all lucky enough to be able to do something like that, but I think that it's nice. Because when you remarry at 45, well, I could still have had children, my gynaecologist was

quite clear about that. He said to me, really, you're not at all menopausal, so… but at 45, no […].

(Isabelle, born in 1941, nurse)

Here, the secondary residence plays a symbolic role for the couple: it represents and consolidates a joint project but is also an element of continuity for the (step) family. This house brings together both families – the children from both sides (Isabelle's and her partner's) – as well as the couple's grandchildren, making it possible to create a sense of family belonging through a fixed point in space.

- So your house in Vaucluse makes these get-togethers possible?
- Yes. Absolutely. That's important. It also brings my husband's children together. He lost his wife, who was of Greek origin, and his Greek brother-in-law came over and spent a week there last summer. So this branch of the family can come to stay with us as well. And there are friends of his wife's who might come this summer. So, you know, we make an effort to preserve the family ties in these… stepfamilies because I think it's important, actually. But, of course, when you have a house in Vaucluse, it's not difficult to get the family together. [It's not like] a house, I don't know, in some remote village where it rains a lot…

We can draw a parallel here with Christophe (Fig. 8.3), who describes his secondary residence in very much the same terms. Christophe married for the first time in 1971 and had a daughter in 1975. He divorced in 1978 and formed a new union in 1981.

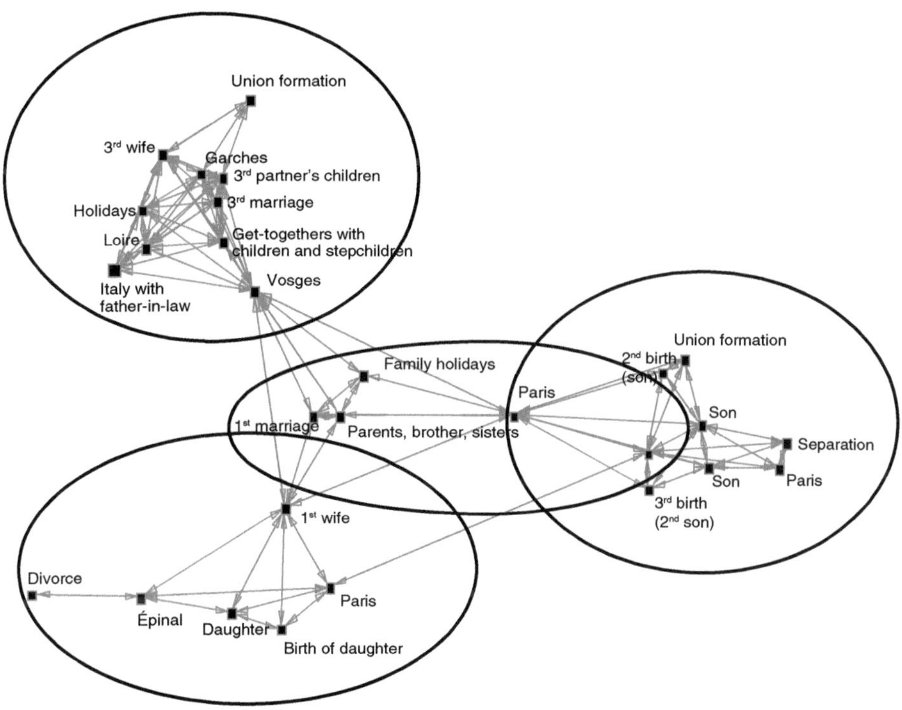

Fig. 8.3 Christophe's family and residential trajectories

He then had two sons with his second partner, and at the same time had custody of his daughter at weekends and during school holidays. In 1987, the couple separated. He moved into an apartment near to his ex-partner in order to stay close to his sons, as well as his daughter. In 1995, he met his third partner and moved in with her in Garches (in the western inner suburbs of Paris), where she lived in an apartment provided by her employer and had custody of her two children. His daughter, now an adult, has never been to this apartment. By contrast, his two sons would come at weekends, and so Christophe built a mezzanine in the living room to accommodate them. Unlike Isabelle, who was reluctant to compare a house to a child, Christophe announces straight away, "It's our baby." The secondary residence is portrayed as a project undertaken as a couple, as a substitute for the child that they have not had together.

> Yes… yes, yes. Let's say that our second home, this is what we said at the time, but we still say it from time to time, it's our baby, because we had our quota of children already and were too old really to have any more, so we invested, we channelled our efforts into something else – this house – because the children, well, they're growing up, they're continuing with their studies, some of them have started… I mean, my eldest has started university, so they're all set to be studying for a while longer, all that kind of thing, so us having a baby together was out of the question, it wasn't worth it, we've got enough on our plates with the ones we've got, so we invested in something else.
> (Christophe, born in 1948, surveyor)

As in Isabelle's case, the secondary residence represents a joint project and "completes" the union: indeed, it was in this residence that the couple married in 2003. It is also the place where the children from each side of the stepfamily come together, even if it is not the only place where certain members of the family meet up, another example being in Italy, where Christophe's current father-in-law lives. However, it is in this secondary residence that all the children from all the various unions are reunited: Christophe's daughter from his first marriage and her daughter (his granddaughter), who are absent from the trips to Italy, come regularly to this secondary residence. For Christophe, it is therefore important to get together with his children in this way.

As he points out:

> Even if I don't live with them, practically all the rest of their time, let's say two thirds of their free time outside school, they spend it with me.

While Agnès Martial (2003) specified the foundational characteristics of the common household, it is not necessarily the primary residence that plays this role, as we have seen. Like the primary residence, the various places frequented by stepfamilies can also be an indicator of the way they function.

Take, for example, Hélène (Fig. 8.4), who applies a totally different rationale. Hélène married at 19. She set up home with her husband in Pontoise (in the north-western outer suburbs of Paris) and had two daughters. The couple bought a house in 1974, and then divorced in 1977. They sold the house and Hélène, who received custody of her two daughters, lived in an apartment that came with her job. In 1987, her second partner moved into her apartment, together with his son. Two years later, the couple separated. Hélène, along with her younger daughter, decided to move, in

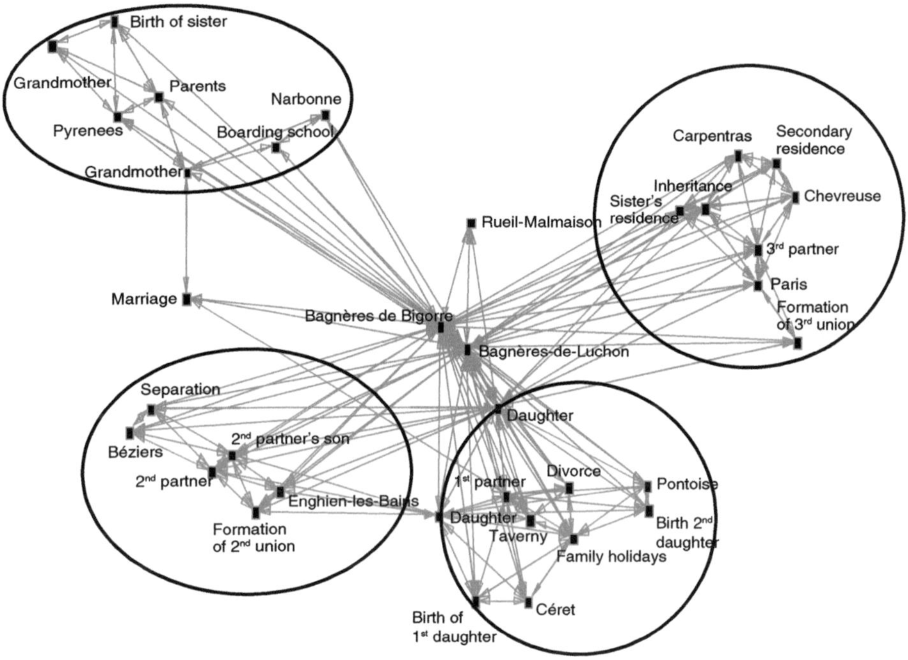

Fig. 8.4 Hélène's family and residential trajectories

order to be closer to her parents in Béziers, in south-western France. However, her daughter's health problems meant she had to return to Paris. It was at this time that she met her third partner, a widower with two children. For 8 years, they each kept their respective dwellings and alternated between them. When Hélène retired, she moved into her partner's home, in Chevreuse (on the south-western fringes of the Paris suburbs).

Unlike Isabelle and Christophe, Hélène did not remarry. However, a system of multiple residences is also in evidence: Hélène inherited her paternal grandmother's house, in Bagnères-de-Bigorre, in the Pyrenees, and bought a house in Bagnères-de-Luchon, a village some 30 miles away where her maternal grandmother lived. These are significant places for Hélène: when she came back from boarding school, she would stay with her grandmothers for the summer holidays. She returns to the area frequently: in the past with her first husband and children, and today with her current partner; they go there every summer. With her partner, Hélène has also bought an apartment in Carpentras, the town in Provence where her elder daughter lives; however, this apartment is not a family undertaking or a place for family get-togethers: it was Hélène who organized all the modernization work and took care of fitting it out and decorating it on her own.

She goes there when she and her partner need some "alone time" away from one another, with her partner staying at the "main residence" in Chevreuse, which does not belong to Hélène (she does not own any part of this property) – a form of intermittent cohabitation observed by Vincent Caradec (1996) among "young older couples", but where it is the second home that marks a "separation" (Gotman et al. 1999) and enables the couple to plan shared time and time alone. So there is a very different logic at work here: the purchase of the apartment was an individual undertaking and does not represent a joint project. It does not fix or symbolize the family made up of the two descent groups: only Hélène's daughters go there. Similarly, other secondary residences are places for the couple and not for the family, which means that the descent groups do not "mix" there. A multi-residence system is in place, but it does not have the same meaning here, as filial ties, while preserved, are above all differentiated. As Hélène points out: "No, just as we have separated our properties, so we have also separated our families."

(Hélène, born in 1943, primary-school teacher)

8.7 Conclusion

This exploratory study of stepfamilies at a different scale – that of domestic and living spaces – has shed light on several points. First of all, adopting a longitudinal perspective and including the various places frequented has highlighted the complexity of conjugal and family trajectories, with some respondents having formed several stepfamilies. However, the existence of several such family sequences does not necessarily lead to the "disappearance" of certain spaces and territories. For example, as we have seen, the paternal family is not excluded, and the paternal grandmother continues to play her role.

This research has also confirmed the role of second homes, most notably as the "symbolic hub where the entire family structure is periodically brought together" (Bonnin and Villanova 1999). At such times, these secondary residences appear to be the centre of family life – serving to reinforce family ties – and the key marker of family identity and history. However, stepfamilies' experience of "fragmented time" (Martial 2003) seems to further encourage the creation of fixed places, in order to bring the family closer together. Indeed, for these families, it would seem that "the secondary residence offers […] a sort of seasonal opportunity to refocus on family life" (Perrot 1998). From this perspective, the secondary residence, like the primary dwelling (Le Gall and Martin 1991), appears to be an indicator of the way a family functions. Accordingly, different approaches have been observed, which make it easier to maintain or strengthen family ties, or even to develop new ones. The family home, often presented as a key part of the family's origins and roots, is a history that has to be invented in the case of stepfamilies: it is linked to a conjugal and family trajectory of which it is the point of origin. Anne Gotman et al. (1999) revealed the dimension of continuity felt by the couple with respect to the second residence, which is considered "one of the sources of accomplishment in one's couple and one's family life" or a means of "revitalizing the conjugal couple". Neither a "new start" nor a "consecration" (Perrot 1998), the second home here signals the start of a commitment to both the conjugal union and the family. It would therefore be interesting to investigate whether stepfamilies' second homes are more often bought or inherited, and whether this affects the way the family functions. After all, the role of a second home is not always to involve the couple in a joint project or to lay down the new roots of a family history; on the contrary, it can be a means of separating not just conjugal territories but also family territories, in particular by associating different dwellings with different descent lines.

References

Barbary, O., & Dureau, F. (1993). Des citadins en mouvement. Analyse des pratiques résidentielles à Quito (Equateur). *Cahiers des Sciences humaines, 29*, 395–418.
Bertaux-Wiame, I. (1995). Familial et résidentiel : un couple indissociable. *Sociologie et sociétés, 2*, 163–175.
Blöss, T. (1997). *Les liens de famille. Sociologie des rapports entre générations*. Paris: PUF.
Blöss, T. (1996). *Éducation familiale et beau-parenté : l'empreinte des trajectoires biographiques*. Paris: L'Harmattan.
Bonnin, P., & de Villanova, R. (1999). *D'une maison à l'autre. Parcours et mobilités résidentielles*. Paris: Créaphis.
Bonvalet, C. (1997). Sociologie de la famille, sociologie du logement un lien à redéfinir. *Sociétés contemporaines, 25*, 25–44.
Bonvalet, C., & Lelièvre, É. (1995). Du concept de ménage à celui d'entourage : une redéfinition de l'espace familial. *Sociologie et sociétés, 2* pp. 177–190.
Burguière, A. (1993). De la famille en miettes à la famille recomposée. In M.-T. Meulders-Klein & I. Théry (Eds.), *Les recompositions familiales aujourd'hui*. Paris: Nathan.
Cadolle, S. (2000). *Être parent, être beau-parent. La recomposition de la famille*. Paris: Éditions Odile Jacob.
Cadolle, S. (2003). *Entraide et solidarités dans les constellations familiales*. Paris: CNAF.
Caradec, V. (1996). Les formes de la vie conjugale des 'jeunes' couples 'âgés'. *Population, 50*(4–5), 897–927.
Clément, C. (2002). *La famille, ruptures et continuités à travers les générations*, sociology and demography thesis supervised by C. Bonvalet, Nanterre Paris-X.
Clément, C. (2009). *La mère et ses enfants. Devenir adulte et transmissions intergénérationnelles*. Paris: L'Harmattan, Coll. Populations.
Courgeau, D. (1975). Le concept de migration. In *Migrations, état civil, recensements administratifs*, actes du 4e colloque de démographie africaine (pp. 27–32). Ouagadougou, 20–24 janvier 1975, Institut national de la statistique et de la démographie.
de Singly, F. (1997). *Habitat et relations familiales*. Paris: Plan Construction et Architecture.
Desplanques, G. (1994). La famille : histoire d'un concept. *Revue française des Affaires sociales, 4*, 95–98.
Flandrin, J.-L. (1984). *Familles. Parenté, maison, sexualité dans l'ancienne société*. Paris: Édition du Seuil.
Frémont, A., Chevalier, J., Hein, R., & Renard, J. (1984). *Géographie sociale*. Paris: Masson.
Gotman, A., et al. (1999). Variations saisonnières de la vie familiale : enquête sur les secondes résidences. In P. Bonnin & R. de Villanova (Eds.), *D'une maison l'autre, parcours et mobilités résidentielles*. Paris: Créaphis.
Le Gall, D. (1996). Beaux-parents au quotidien et par intermittence. In D. Le Gall & C. Martin (Eds.), *Familles et politiques sociales. Dix questions sur le lien familial contemporain*. Paris: L'Harmattan.
Le Gall, D., & Martin, C. (1988a). *Le réseau de parenté après la désunion*. Paris: CNAF.

Le Gall, D., & Martin, C. (1988b). Le réseau parental après un divorce ou une séparation. *Dialogue, 101*, 85–93.
Le Gall, D., & Martin, C. (1991). *Recomposition familiale et usage de l'espace domestique*. Paris: Plan Construction et Architecture.
Le Gall, D., & Martin, C. (1993). Transitions familiales, logiques de recomposition et modes de régulation conjugale. In M.-T. Meulders-Klein & I. Théry (Eds.), *Les recompositions familiales aujourd'hui*. Paris: Nathan.
Martial, A. (2003). *S'apparenter. Ethnologie des liens de familles recomposées*. Paris: Éditions de la Maison des sciences de l'homme.
Perrot, M. (1998). La maison de famille. In Dubost F. (Ed.) L'autre maison. La résidence secondaire, refuge des générations. *Autrement*, 178.
Pinson, D. (1988). *Du logement pour tous aux maisons en tous genres*. Paris: Plan Construction et Architecture, coll. Recherches.
Poittevin, A. (2003). *Les liens dans les fratries recomposées*, Dossiers d'études. Allocations familiales, 47.
Théry, I. (1987). Remariage et familles recomposées : des évidences aux incertitudes. *L'année sociologique, 37*, 119–152.
Théry, I. (1991). Trouver le mot juste. Langage et parenté dans les recompositions familiales après divorce. In M. Segalen (Ed.), *Jeux de famille*. Paris: CNRS Éditions.
Théry, I. (1996). (1st edition 1993). *Le démariage. Justice et vie privée.* Paris: Odile Jacob.

Chapter 9
Family Places

Catherine Bonvalet and Éva Lelièvre

Considering the space in which kinship ties are organized has become one of the most fruitful approaches to studying the way in which the contemporary family functions. As early as the mid-1970s, Catherine Gokalp and Louis Roussel showed the surprising residential proximity that existed between parents and their adult children. Since then, numerous studies have confirmed that the family extends well beyond the nucleus to include several generations outside the domestic group (Attias-Donfut 1995). Similarly, in spatial terms, families are not rooted to the single fixed point that is the primary residence (Pinson 1988; Bonnin and de Villanova 1999). In order to understand the relationships between families and spaces, some researchers have therefore sought to challenge the classic notion of household, with its attendant limitations. Instead, they propose other concepts such as the *entourage* and the *residential system* (Dureau 2002). The concept of entourage aims to broaden the reference group of a given individual by taking account of non-co-resident children, life partners and siblings, as well as all those people with whom individuals have co-resided at some point in their life (Bonvalet and Lelièvre 1995; Lelièvre et al. 1998). The concept of residential system is defined as the configuration of places that include the residences of the individuals' relatives and close friends on the one hand, and secondary residences on the other. The idea that the place of residence is not the only point of reference for a given individual is nothing new, and indeed can be traced back to the emergence of the notion of life spaces[1] (Chevalier 1974; Frémont et al. 1984; Courgeau 1975; Rosental 1993).

This article initially appeared in the journal *Espaces et sociétés*, 2005, 1–2, pp. 99–122.

[1] "Life space" is defined as "the space frequented by each of us, with its attractive places and hubs around which an individual's experience is constructed: the dwelling, the home, places of work and leisure, etc. This is the tangible space of day-to-day life" – see A. Frémont, J. Chevalier, R. Hein and J. Renard, 1984; see also G. Di Méo, 1991.

C. Bonvalet (✉) • É. Lelièvre (✉)
Institut national d'études démographiques (INED), Paris, France
e-mail: bonvalet@ined.fr; eva@ined.fr

C. Bonvalet, É. Lelièvre (eds.), *Family Beyond Household and Kin*,
INED Population Studies 6, DOI 10.1007/978-3-319-24684-0_9

All these approaches aim to capture the multiple ways in which individuals are located in space, and their movements between different places, especially those associated with the family. More specifically, these approaches focus on movements between multiple dwellings belonging to members of the kinship group. Over time, a residential system develops which characterize the group of people linked in this way. In a context where family ties are no longer determined in advance by position in the family tree (son of …, father of…, sister of…, etc.) but have become increasingly elective, the way in which the family organizes its territory by becoming concentrated in one place – or, conversely, by remaining dispersed in space – provides an indication of the ties between relatives. Individuals shape their entourage of family and close friends through interplay of distance and proximity. Studying the way in which spaces are associated with the dynamics of affinity involves analysing the relationships that people maintain with members of their "chosen" family, as geographical proximity helps to construct social ties by facilitating face-to-face contact (Bonvalet et al. 2007).

Numerous studies have focused on families' relationship with space, primarily with respect to places of origin, beginning with the places of birth of respondents and respondents' parents (Pourcher 1964; Bonvalet 1987), which for Anne Gotman constitute the reference and foundational spaces when they also correspond to places of childhood and adolescence (Gotman 2007). Research on the spatial distribution of relatives forms a second line of study that led to the geographical mapping of the family (Lebras and Goré 1985) and highlighted the ways in which families organize themselves in spatial terms (Roussel and Bourguignon 1976; Gokalp 1978; Bonvalet 1991; Lelièvre and Imbert 2002). More recently, research has shown that this grouping can take place outside the primary residence, and more particularly within the secondary residence (Dubost 1998; Bonnin and de Villanova 1999). This secondary residence is often the focus of both emotional and financial investment. As Françoise Dubost writes: "Secondary residents should not be confused with tourists or holidaymakers. They live, reside and are rooted in a given place."

The analysis of relationships between families and housing has thus been pursued by investigating whether family types can be characterized by their relations and attitudes to housing and space. The aim here was not to recreate a typology of families or domestic groups based on co-residence and the community of property, as in Le Play or Laslett (1972), but rather to see whether a residential system formed by the location of the residences of all family members corresponded to a particular "family space". For just as the domestic group – in other words, the household – is defined and described in terms of dwellings, so the location of related persons within the same geographical area makes it possible to define and analyse the composition of family groups comprising several households. Peter Willmott's (1987) classification of such groups into "local extended families", "dispersed extended families" and "attenuated extended families" represented an initial line of research, which we pursued in the *Proches et parents* survey by differentiating between "local family entourages", characterized by strong residential proximity and intense relationships, and "dispersed family entourages" (Bonvalet and Maison 2007).[2]

In this chapter, we seek to establish links between these different studies by examining in turn "theoretical map of family places", based first on places of origin and places of kinship, subsequently complemented by a map of places which are regularly visited by respondents, such as second homes or other regularly frequented places.

Our objective, therefore, is to broaden an analysis that, rather than describing the "life space"[3] of the individuals surveyed, instead describes the "family life space" constituted by all "family places" mobilized; the aim is not to juxtapose these spaces or study them independently, but rather to determine their respective positions in the patterns of behaviours of respondents and their entourages.

9.1 From Life Spaces to Family Territories

The *Biographies et entourage* survey by INED collected data about the family, residential and occupational trajectories of 2830 people aged 50–70 (birth cohorts born between 1930 and 1950) residing in the Paris region,[4] as well as the trajectories of members of their entourage.[5] Using the mosaic of places that make up the geographical universe of each respondent, we shall gradually build up a picture of how a given family territory is constructed.

In this first approach to family territories, we propose a number of simple definitions. The relevant data was collected with a view to analysing several forms of territories: territories of origin, territories covered in the past, territories frequented at the time of the survey, and planned future territories. The detailed information thus obtained (Lelièvre et al. 1998) can be used to reconstruct the different geographical universes that succeed one another throughout respondents' lives.

One of the most important choices we first made was to select only those places with links to the family – hereafter referred to as "family places" – to the

[2] We had defined the "local family entourage" using four criteria: affinities (relatives designated as close); frequency of contact (at least once a week); mutual assistance (the close relative has been helped by the respondent, or vice versa); and residential proximity (living in the same or a neighbouring *commune* [municipality]).

[3] Namely, according to Daniel Courgeau's (1980) definition, "the portion of space where an individual conducts all his or her activities […] not only those places where an individual stays or passes through, but also all those places with which the individual interacts".

[4] The Paris region comprises the city and *département* of Paris and the seven surrounding *départements* (Hauts-de-Seine, Seine-Saint-Denis, Val-de-Marne, Essonne, Yvelines, Val-d'Oise, Seine-et-Marne).

[5] In addition to detailed descriptions concerning a varied universe of people and places, each questionnaire systematically collected data on the familial, occupational and residential trajectories of 2830 respondents and those of their parents and partners, representing some 11,000–12,000 interconnected life histories in all.

Table 9.1 Selected places within the family network

Relationship	Places of birth	Places of residence	Places frequented[a]	Secondary residences
Ascendants				
Maternal and paternal grandparents	X			
Biological and adoptive parents	X	X		
Respondent	X	X	X	X
Collateral relatives				
Siblings and half-siblings		X		
Descendants				
Respondent's children		X		
Partner's children		X		

Source: *Biographies et entourage* survey, INED, 2001
[a]Only places relating to the family were included here

exclusion of all places relating to work, leisure or shopping. Similarly, places frequented on holiday that were not family residences were also excluded. Furthermore, the contours of the family that we highlight here are limited to the descent group, i.e. the respondent's parents, siblings and children (in the broadest sense, as children of respondents' partners are included here).[6] Finally, only those places inhabited or frequented at the time of the survey have been considered. The survey date therefore represents a point in time to which previous situations (measurable via the information collected in the survey) can then be compared in order to trace the changes in this territory throughout the lifetimes of the individuals surveyed.

Table 9.1 presents all the places selected in this chapter. Depending on whether we are talking about rootedness or territory, or referring to places of origin or territories that are known, crossed or frequented at a given moment in time, the described space varies, providing different perspectives on how the family network interacts with space.

A number of complementary aspects of family territories shall also be explored:

- origins, via the places of birth of ascendants, which is particularly useful for considering rootedness;
- the range of possibilities offered by the places of residence of members of the descent group;
- finally, the frequented family places where respondents regularly spend time or reside.

[6]Only relatives who were alive at the time of the survey.

In addition, the survey, restricted to residents of the Paris region, enables us to describe the territorial configurations of this region's inhabitants at the time of the survey.

9.2 The Territory of the Family… in Terms of Origins

Ever since the work of Jacques Bertillon (1894), the origins of Parisians have been widely studied by researchers, in particular by Louis Chevalier (1950) who examined the formation of the Parisian population and Guy Pourcher (1964) who focused on the population distribution of Paris. Our analysis of the origins of residents of the Paris region is consistent with previous findings: 40 % of respondents were born in the Paris region (compared with 43 % in the *Peuplement et dépeuplement de Paris* survey). The rest are, for the most part, originally from provincial France (35 %) or from abroad (24 %). Only 1.5 % were born in French overseas *départements* and territories. Those respondents born abroad were mostly from North Africa (23.7 % from Algeria, 11 % from Morocco and 6.7 % from Tunisia) and Southern Europe (14.6 % from Portugal, 4.5 % from Italy and 4 % from Spain). For the 1926–1935 birth cohorts in the *Peuplement et dépeuplement de Paris*[7] survey and the 1930–1950 cohorts in the *Biographies et entourage* survey, migrants from Brittany, Normandy, Picardy and the far north of France represented 35 % of all provincial respondents in both surveys.

However, place of birth alone is not enough to establish ties between respondents and their region of origin. For example, this tie may be very weak for respondents whose parents lived in the area for only a short period around the time of their birth, or, on the contrary, very strong if several generations have lived there and continue to do so. These ties therefore depend upon the rootedness and attachment of the family to the region of birth. One way of studying these ties without pre-empting their actual strength is to include the origins of respondents' parents and grandparents in the analysis of their origins.

If we consider only individuals who live in the city of Paris proper, around one respondent in five was born there. Among these respondents born in Paris – a small minority of all respondents – half have at least one parent who was also born in Paris and 20 % have two Parisian-born parents (this latter group represents an extremely low proportion of all residents of the city of Paris of these generations).

If we now consider all respondents born in the Paris region, almost two thirds have at least one parent who was also born there, and 26 % have two parents born in this region (corresponding to around 1 in 10 of all respondents).

[7] The *Biographies et entourage* survey continues the lines of study explored by other INED surveys, and more specifically the following: *Peuplement de Paris* in 1960 by Guy Pourcher among the 1901–1910 birth cohorts, *Triple biographie* in 1981 by Daniel Courgeau among the 1911–1935 birth cohorts, and *Peuplement et dépeuplement de Paris* in 1986 by Catherine Bonvalet among the 1926–1935 birth cohorts (see Chap. 2).

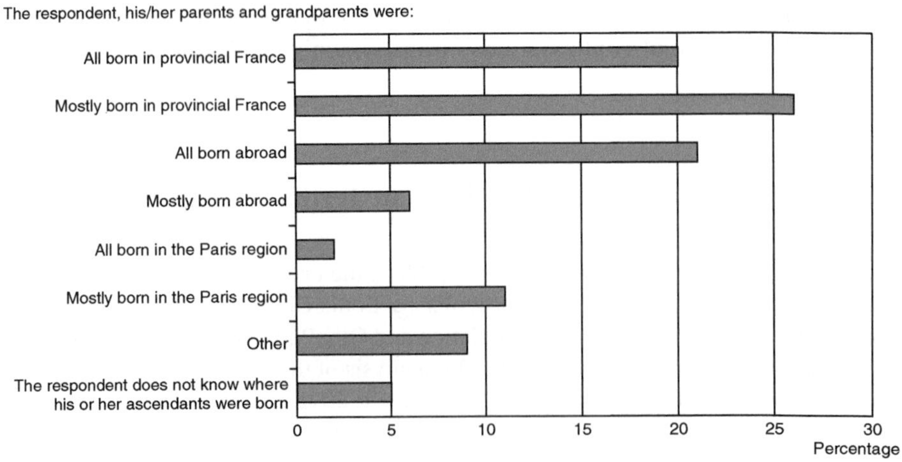

Fig. 9.1 Configuration of respondents' origins (*Source*: *Biographies et entourage* survey, INED, 2001)

Figure 9.1 shows the proportion of persons (among respondent + parents + grandparents, i.e. seven people in total) who were born, respectively, in provincial France, in the Paris region, and abroad. In all, 20 % of the 2830 respondents are of exclusively provincial origin (i.e. all seven members of the group were born in provincial France). If we also include those respondents whose ascendants are mostly of provincial origin, a total of 46 % of all respondents are concerned.

Respondents whose ascendants were mostly foreign-born represent 27 % of the total sample. Finally, 13 % of respondents have ascendants who were born exclusively or mostly in the Paris region (2 % and 11 % of the sample, respectively). In terms of lineage, therefore, only a minority of respondents are truly rooted in the Paris region.

9.3 The Territory of the Entourage… at the Time of the Survey

The territory of the current family entourage of Paris region residents can be delimited by considering the places of residence of the respondents' parents, siblings and children. This is a space defined exclusively by the location of the family, regardless of how often these places are actually frequented.

On average, these entourages contain six people, and over half of respondents have a family entourage comprising three to six individuals. Respondents with entourages of more than ten people are rare. Small entourages primarily concern the oldest respondents (aged 65 and over), a majority of whom are female.

9.3.1 The Residential Proximity of Family Members

Residential proximity is an important element that shapes the territories of the family entourage. The residential configuration formed by the places of residence of the ascendants, siblings and descendants of respondents (who were aged 50–70 at the time of the survey) derives from the sum of all individual trade-offs within the descent group. Geographical proximity or distance are the product of complex phenomena determined by factors such as the occupational and family constraints of members of the respondent's entourage on the one hand, and ties that may have developed between people and places in which they have lived on the other. Proximity and distance can both be the result of either a choice to spend time together with family members or, on the contrary, a desire to distance oneself from family life. Both, however, can be experienced as involuntary in situations where individuals feel they are imprisoned by their family (Gotman 1999) or, conversely, obliged to move away. Accordingly, the space we observe at the time of the survey can be interpreted to a certain extent as the "best" possible arrangement for accommodating the different ways in which each family functions; it reflects the trade-offs between constraints and aspirations in a relational universe characterized by affinities and enmities.

Table 9.2 indicates the proportions of people who actually live close to a member of their family in the Paris region. Whether this is the result of a real choice or merely for reasons of convenience, it should be remembered that living in the same *commune*[8] as one or more relatives (or a neighbouring *commune*) means being part of a relational space that facilitates access to family resources. As a result, access to housing in these places is no doubt easier.

Almost one family in six (among families where not all are co-resident) have at least two members who live in the same *département*.[9] If we consider only those respondents born in the Paris region, these proportions are significantly higher in each case.

The greatest residential proximity is found between respondents' households and those of their children (55 % live in the same *département* as one of their children), of one of their siblings (31 % of respondents), or, lastly, of one of their parents. Whether a respondent lives in the same *commune* or *département* as his/her parents depends to a large extent on his or her migration trajectory. Geographical clustering tends to be observed among provincial or foreign respondents and their siblings or children, whereas the parents often remain in their province or country of birth. For respondents born in the Paris region, proximity with parents is

---

[8] A *commune* is a municipality with an elected mayor and council. French *communes* vary enormously in size, ranging from small villages with a handful of residents to large cities with populations in the hundreds of thousands.

[9] A *département* is a middle-tier administrative division (between the *commune* and the region) that is roughly equivalent to an English county. France is currently divided into 101 *départements*, five of which are overseas.

Table 9.2 Spatial distribution of relatives of respondents in the *Biographies et Entourage* survey (%)

	Same *commune*	Same or neighbouring *commune*	Same *département*	Number concerned
Mother or father	9	19	22	1312
Respondents born in Paris region	16	34	41	500
Respondents born outside Paris region	4	9	10	812
At least one child	25	45	55	2071
Respondents born in Paris region	27	47	57	833
Respondents born outside Paris region	24	44	53	1238
At least one child of a partner	7	24	29	314
Respondents born in Paris region	5	22	29	125
Respondents born outside Paris region	9	25	29	190
At least one brother or sister	11	26	31	2387
Respondents born in Paris region	18	37	45	875
Respondents born outside Paris region	6	20	22	1512
At least one parent or child	22	40	47	2830
Respondents born in Paris region	26	45	54	1129
Respondents born outside Paris region	20	36	43	1701
At least one member of the family	27	50	58	2830
Respondents born in Paris region	33	57	66	1129
Respondents born outside Paris region	23	45	53	1701

Source: *Biographies et entourage* survey, INED, 2001

equivalent to that observed with siblings, but is still more than 10 % lower than the levels of proximity between respondents and their children.

If we now consider a more detailed geographical level – namely the *commune* of residence – a remarkable level of stability is observed: half of all families living in the Paris region take advantage of the socialization that comes with residential proximity. It is striking to note the high level of rootedness of respondents' families in this extremely urbanized region whose population distribution is largely the result of extensive inward migration. Even in France's largest metropolitan area, the family is not isolated, and this observation – revealed by past studies and confirmed 15 years ago for the 1926–1935 birth cohorts (Bonvalet 1991) – remains true for the geographical locations of descent groups of the 1930–1950 birth cohorts surveyed in 2000–2001.

9.3.2 The Place of the Paris Region in These Territories

The territorial configuration of these families can take various forms depending on the size of the family network and the number of regions concerned. Certain families are based solely in the Paris region, while others have members in provincial

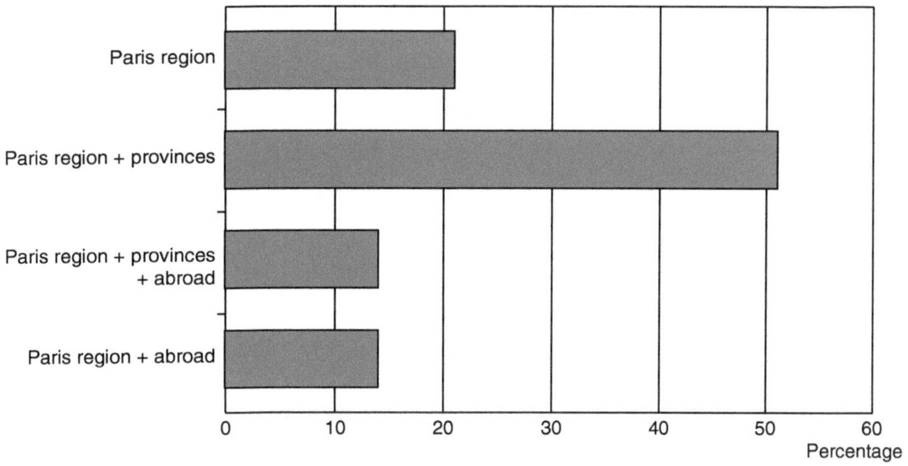

Fig. 9.2 Configuration of family territories (*Source*: *Biographies et entourage* survey, INED, 2001)

France and others extend to nearby or distant countries. An entourage divided between the Paris region and other regions of France is by far the most common residential configuration (half of all respondents). These family networks include five people on average (Fig. 9.2).

A minority of entourages (21 %) are based entirely in the Paris region. These family networks are also much smaller than those of other respondents, with an average size of three people.

For all other respondents (28 %, i.e. more than one in four), the territory of the family entourage is split between the Paris region, other regions of France, other countries or French overseas *départements* and territories, or exclusively in the Paris region and other countries. These respondents tend to reside in the centre of the Paris region and over a third are foreign-born. Typically, their siblings and parents still live abroad; the members of their entourage who live in the Paris region tend to be their children and also often a sibling. At individual level, however the respondents' situations are highly diverse.

Specific examples are presented in Figs. 9.3 and 9.4 to illustrate the most common configurations of family territories.

Depending on the number of regions over which the family network is spread, and their location with respect to the Paris region (e.g. nearby in the case of the Eure *département* but far away in the case of the respondent with family members in the Aveyron, Bas-Rhin and Seine-Maritime *départements*), families' territories differ in shape and extent.

The same diversity exists for family networks whose territories extend into both provincial France and other countries. This is not just a question of considering two "clusters" – one in provincial France and the other abroad, typically in the respondent's country of origin – but also of more complex configurations that reflect both the respondent's trajectory and the trajectories of the respondent's siblings and children.

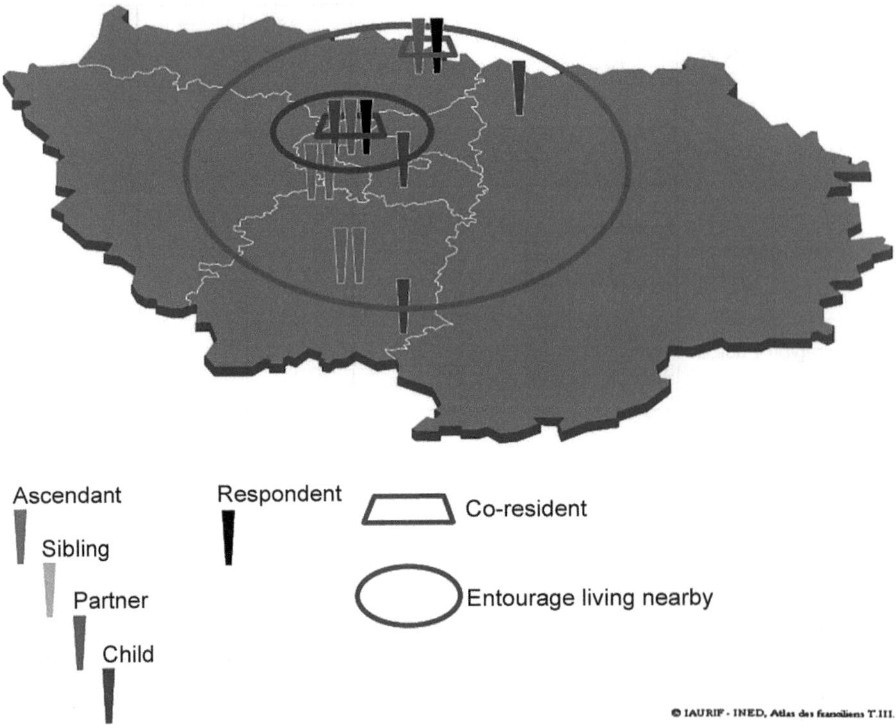

Fig. 9.3 Regional spread of family territories. Two examples of entourages with "Paris region" configurations. *Interpretation*: the respondent's entourage is composed of the ascendants, siblings, partner and children of the respondent at the time of the survey. Some of these family members might live in the same dwelling as the respondent (i.e. they are co-resident), others might live in a different dwelling nearby (i.e. within the Paris region), while others might live farther away (in other regions of France, in French overseas *départements* and territories, or abroad) (*Source*: *Biographies et entourage* survey, INED, 2001)

9.3.3 The Regional Diversity of These Territories

Beyond the distinction between the Paris region and the rest of a family's territory, it is useful to consider the places where members of the descent group live, whether they are grouped together or spread out, forming different clusters within the respondent's life space (centred on his or her residence in the Paris region). Table 9.3a shows the distribution of family territories by the number of different regions[10] where their relatives live, whatever the size of the family network, while

[10] Twenty-two regions are considered: Paris region (Île-de-France), Champagne-Ardenne, Picardy, Upper Normandy, Centre-Val de Loire, Lower Normandy, Burgundy, Nord–Pas-de-Calais, Lorraine, Alsace, Franche-Comté, Pays de la Loire, Brittany, Poitou-Charentes, Aquitaine, Midi-Pyrénées, Limousin, Rhône-Alpes, Auvergne, Languedoc-Roussillon, Provence-Alpes-Côte d'Azur, Corsica.

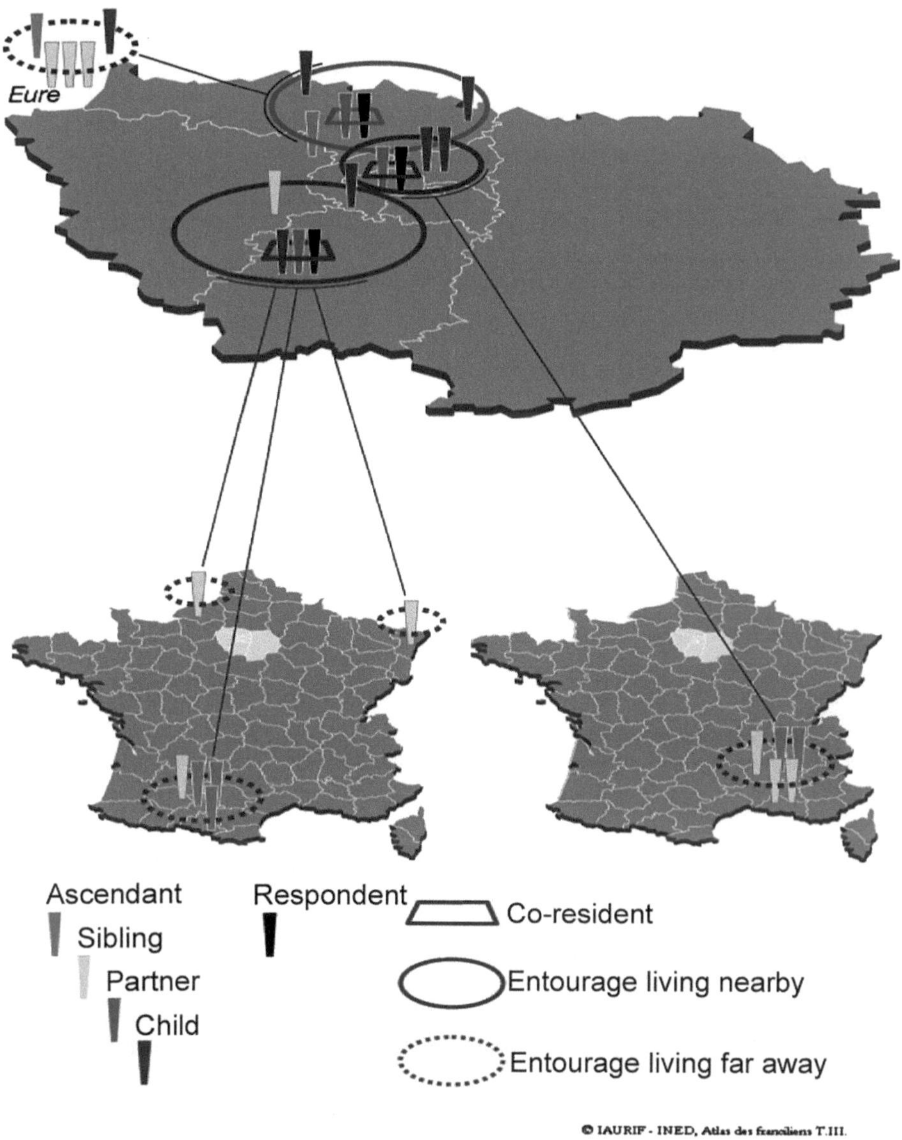

Fig. 9.4 Regional spread of family territories. Three examples of entourages with "Paris region + provinces" configurations (*Interpretation and source*: see Fig. 9.3)

Table 9.3b presents this same distribution for different sizes of family network, as this size factor inevitably affects the geographical spread of family networks.

Around half of respondents have family networks covering just one or two regions, while only 18 % have networks with more complex regional diversity involving four regions or more. If we now consider these same distributions while

Table 9.3a Regional dispersion[a] of family territories

	None	1 region	2 regions	3 regions	4 regions	5 regions	6+ regions
%	–	21.7	35.3	25.5	11.2	4.6	1.7
Number	16	611	993	717	316	129	48
Distribution in regions excluding the Paris region							
%	15.2	38.3	27.1	13.0	5.0	1.4	–
Number	428	1080	763	366	140	40	13

Source: *Biographies et entourage* survey, INED, 2001
[a]This distribution excludes the respondent's place of residence (which is necessarily in the Paris region)

Table 9.3b Regional dispersion[a] of family territories by network size

	1 region	2 region	3 regions	4 regions	5 regions	6+ regions
4-person family network						
%	27.8	45.7	22.5	4.0		
Number	131	215	106	19		
6-person family network						
%	12.3	33.4	34.6	16.1	3.0	–
Number	51	139	144	67	14	1
8-person family network						
%	7.0	26.6	31.4	18.1	12.8	4.0
Number	16	60	71	41	29	9

Source: *Biographies et entourage* survey, INED, 2001
[a]This distribution excludes the respondent's place of residence (which is necessarily in the Paris region)

excluding the Paris region, it becomes clear that the vast majority of respondents have links, via their families, with provincial France or other countries (2402 individuals, or 85 % of all respondents). Once the Paris region is removed from the mix, regional diversity is much lower, with only 6 % of respondents having family networks spread across four regions or more.

However, as only networks comprising at least four people can potentially extend over four regions (or more), it is useful to examine the territorial spread for a given network size.

In fact, it is only for family networks with six members or more that the regional dispersion (including the Paris region) becomes more pronounced, with 19 % of these families spread over at least four different regions, rising to 30 % for family networks comprising eight individuals.

9.4 Places of Family Rootedness

The family geography we have described so far provides information about *all* places of residence of family members that may potentially figure in respondents' networks of family spaces – a "map" of possibilities or, to put it another way, a

Table 9.4 Places frequented (distribution of all places cited by respondents)

Places frequented	Number	Percentage
Family	1113	59
Friends	242	13
Respondent	17	1
Partner	52	3
Other[a]	362	20
Not declared	67	4
Total	1853	100

Source: *Biographies et entourage* survey, INED, 2001

[a]"Other" typically corresponds to regions or countries that respondents frequented as a child but for which no particular family member was cited

background map over which respondents can then trace their actual networks. The information collected by the *Biographies et entourage* survey also allows us to analyse all residences that are regularly frequented, whether these are second homes or other family residences. However, the spaces described above, defined by the places of residence in respondents' family networks, have not been taken account of any criteria relating to the frequency of respondents' visits.[11] We have therefore decided to examine and compare information collected by different means, where respondents directly identified those places that they actually frequented.[12]

9.4.1 Places Frequented

Of all the places frequented regularly at the time of the survey (1853 places in all), family places were by far the most common (Table 9.4). Only 13 % were dwellings belonging to friends, while 20 % were holiday destinations to which respondents returned every year (either to campsites or to rented accommodation). Some of these dwellings, while owned by respondents, were not, however, defined as secondary residences; they represent a small minority of cases (less than 1 %), and typically reflect a different kind of investment.[13] Similarly, we observed that few respondents reported regularly frequenting their partner's second homes which they had not declared as second home. Two possible reasons for this can be considered: the first

[11]These places are recorded in the context of questions relating to the locations, occupations and marital statuses of members of respondents' families.

[12]The questions were worded as follows: "We would now like to talk about other places that you have frequented throughout your lifetime. As an adult, have you acquired a second home? At present, what other places do you regularly frequent or have an attachment to?" In this article, we have considered only those places with links to respondents' families.

[13]These include multi-owner properties in seaside or ski resorts (i.e. timeshares). In these cases, the respondent has access to these properties for only 1 or 2 weeks per year.

Table 9.5 Number of respondents who frequent places other than their primary residence (distribution by number of places)

Number of residences	Number of respondents with access to other family residences	Percentage
One	619	71
Two	186	21
Three	52	6
Four or more	21	2
Total	878	100

Source: *Biographies et entourage* survey, INED, 2001

is that the partner acquired this dwelling as part of an inheritance and the respondent feels no attachment to it; the second is that the respondent forms part of a stepfamily where each partner keeps their own property.[14] We have chosen to include all places belonging to the family or family-in-law.

Under these criteria, 1249 dwellings belonging to family members corresponded to places frequented by our respondents from the Paris region. We observed that they were very unevenly distributed, as only one respondent in three (878 individuals in total) regularly stayed in a family dwelling (Table 9.5). With this in mind, the average number of dwellings frequented, not counting second homes, was 1.42, with a minority having access to three or four family-owned homes (the maximum recorded was nine dwellings).

These places can take diverse forms: family homes that belong to grandparents or were inherited by parents or an aunt or uncle, primary or secondary residences of a family member, or timeshare apartments in seaside or ski resorts.

As people are living longer, a large number of respondents still have at least one living parent (46 %). This proportion increases if we also include partners' parents. Bearing in mind that only 22 % of respondents live in the same *département* as their parents and just under 40 % live in the same region (Paris region), most respondents find themselves spending time in provincial France or abroad to visit their parents, be it for holidays, family reunions or to help and support their parents in the event of illness or dependence. The importance of the support provided by adult children to their elderly parents has been clearly established for these same generations (Attias-Donfut 1995; Ortalda 2001). This assistance, especially in the domestic realm, is typically centred on the parent(s)' home, often requiring travel, in some case over long distances if they do not live in the Paris area. It is not surprising, therefore, to observe that parents' primary or secondary residences represent 41 % of first-cited family places (Table 9.6). Next in the list are siblings' residences (almost one in five cases, including partners' siblings). The extended family – including aunts and uncles, cousins, and nieces and nephews – are also well represented (almost 18 % of first-cited places visited).

[14] See Chap. 8.

Table 9.6 Places frequented (distribution of family places cited by respondents) (%)

	First place cited	Second place cited	All places cited
Parents	25.4	12.7	20.8
Partner's parents	15.7	12.7	13.4
Children or partner's children	8.4	15.1	10.4
Sibling	14.5	24.7	19.4
Partner's sibling	4.2	5.4	4.9
Aunt or uncle	3.8	2.3	3.9
Family	15.2	13.1	13.6
Partner's family	2.7	1.6	2.6
Respondent	1.5	1.5	1.4
Partner	5.1	2.7	4.2
Other[a]	4.5	8.1	5.4
Number	*878*	*259*	*1249*

Source: *Biographies et entourage survey,* INED, 2001
[a]"Other" typically corresponds to regions or countries that respondents frequented as a child but for which no particular family member was cited

Respondents' children's places, by contrast, are quite rarely cited and only when they have left the Paris region for other regions or moved abroad. In these cases, respondents spend time at their children's home, in particular to see their grandchildren. The number of visits to children remains low in comparison to the significant proportion of respondents concerned – in all, 45 % of respondents with adult offspring have at least one child who lives outside the Paris region. The relatively low proportion of visits can be explained by the fact that family reunions often take place at the homes of respondents or their parents. It seems that parents' residences often remain family places, while children's residences more rarely obtain this status (Table 9.6).

9.4.2 Secondary Residences: Continuity or Creation of a Family Place

In the *Biographies et entourage* survey, 36 % of respondents owned at least one secondary residence (almost 4 % owned at least two[15]). In total, 1119 secondary residences were recorded, owned by 1006 households (Table 9.7). As the individuals interviewed were 50–70 years old, it is not surprising to observe a high percentage of second homeowners – after all, it is at this age that residential plans start to

[15] Secondary residences make up only a small part of households' property assets. According to the 2002 *Logement* (Housing) survey, secondary residences only represented 31 % of retirees' property assets and 29 % of those of working-age respondents over 50, with rental properties accounting for more than half of the total. The ownership rate for other dwellings varies by social class: it is higher among craft workers, farmers and executives, and lower among office and manual workers (Minodier and Rieg 2004).

Table 9.7 Number of respondents who own a secondary residence

Number of residences	One	Two	Three or more	Total
Number of respondents who are homeowners	906	90	10	1006
Percentage	90	9	1	100

Source: *Bibliographies et entourage* survey, INED, 2001

be less concerned with the primary residence (either because the individuals have already purchased and paid off their first home, or, in the case of tenants, because they wish to invest in property via a second home); it is also at this age that inheritances come into the equation, following the deaths of parents and parents-in-law.

The Paris region is characterized by a higher proportion of secondary homeowners than other regions. The 2002 *Logement* survey clearly shows that while retiree households are less likely to be owners of their primary residence, they are more likely to own a secondary dwelling (Minodier and Rieg 2004). As house prices in the Paris region are high, a certain number of households are discouraged from buying in the region and so fulfil their desires to become homeowners by acquiring a secondary residence. Many recent studies have shown the importance of the secondary residence, which is often secondary only in name (Remy 1995; Bonnin and de Villanova 1999). Indeed, this additional home frequently plays an essential role in the way the family functions: it is the place where parents, children, grandparents and grandchildren get together, far from day-to-day constraints (Bonvalet 1991), and the venue *par excellence* for family reunions, especially in the case of migrants (Bonnin and de Villanova 1999) or stepfamilies (see Chap. 8). What we see here – and what we previously observed in the *Peuplement et dépeuplement de Paris* survey – is the wholesale relocation of the family "centre" to the coast, the mountains and the countryside. The process is multiform: one family member moves to a particular place and invites their siblings to spend their holidays there. A family home is inherited, a piece of land or a property comes up for sale and is bought by another family member; alternatively, to ensure that everyone retains their independence, someone buys a small house close to their elderly parents, and their siblings do the same, etc.

The importance of grandchildren is very apparent in the strategies for buying or securing a second home. Respondents who have grandchildren are slightly more likely to have a secondary residence than those who have no grandchildren (38 % compared to 33 %). Some build an additional bedroom; others devote a room or a corner of the house to their grandchildren so that they feel at home when they visit, with their own bed and toy box (over half of respondents who are both grandparents and homeowners have a specific bedroom or space for their grandchildren): "The house then fulfils its role: to bring the family together under the same roof" (Bonvalet 1991).

However, alongside this very "intimate" or "close-knit" configuration of the family, other practices relating to secondary residences – described by Anne Gotman and Jean-Michel Léger – also exist, namely the desire for dispersal, where the various family members go about their own business in distinct territories, and in

Table 9.8 Distribution of respondents by type of family place frequented

	Number of places concerned		Number of respondents concerned relative to the total sample		
	Number	%	Number	%	%
Secondary residences	1119	47	1006	62	36
Family places frequented	1249	53	878	54	31
Total	2368	100	1619	[a]	57

Source: *Biographies et entourage* survey, INED, 2001
[a]The number of individuals who frequent at least one place is not equal to the sum of individuals who own a secondary residence and those who frequent an additional place, as certain respondents are both secondary homeowners and frequent another family place

processes of separation, where the secondary residence gradually becomes the preferred place of one partner while the other occupies the primary residence.[16] In this case, the residence in question is no longer a place for family get-togethers but a place taken over by successive generations, or even partners.

But multi-residence practices are not restricted to the respondent's secondary residence. Secondary residences represent just 47 % of all the family places frequented by Paris region residents, even if, in terms of the households concerned, secondary homeowners represent 62 % of the individuals who benefit from access to another dwelling in addition to their main residence (Table 9.8). Over half of all Paris region residents in this age range (50–70 years in 2000) have at least one other place they can go to on a regular basis.

In total, 57 % of respondents regularly go to family properties belonging either to themselves or their parents (Table 9.9). For 39 % of all respondents, this family place is the only such place frequented, and is typically a secondary residence (24 %, compared with 15 % for family dwellings). Nevertheless, owning a secondary residence does not prevent households from moving between different places (10 % of all respondents). A quarter of households who own a secondary residence frequent at least one other family place in addition to this residence. If we include all secondary residences and places frequented – 2368 dwellings in total – respondents have access to an average of 1.46 family dwellings. However, if we consider all residents of the Paris region, this figure falls to less than one dwelling on average (0.8).

This means that certain households have substantial family real-estate assets, while others have no residential resources other than their primary residence (43 % of Paris region residents).

In the vast majority of cases, these assets are located outside the Paris region – only 5 % of these dwellings are located in the Paris urban area. The key function of

[16]This is also the case with stepfamilies where each partner wishes to keep a home for themselves where they can accommodate their own children and grandchildren in a context that remains separate from the new partner's family. See, for example, the case of Isabelle in Chap. 8.

Table 9.9 Distribution of respondents among the different types of residences frequented

Respondents with *n* secondary residences	Number of respondents by number of places belonging to the family: None	One	Two	Three	Four	Five or more	Total
No secondary residence (number)	1211	426	133	42	7	5	1824
(%)	42.79	15.05	4.70	1.48	0.25	0.18	64.45
One (number)	667	177	46	9	4	3	906
(%)	23.57	6.25	1.63	0.32	0.14	0.07	32.01
Two (number)	66	14	7	1	1	1	90
(%)	2.33	0.49	0.25	0.04	0.04	0.04	3.18
Three or more (number)	8	2	0	0	0	0	10
(%)	0.29	0.07	0.00	0.00	0.00	0.00	0.36
Total (number)	1952	619	186	52	12	9	2830
(%)	68.98	21.87	6.57	1.84	0.42	0.18	100.00

Source: *Biographies et entourage* survey, INED, 2001

Table 9.10 Distribution of respondents by number of different regions frequented

	Number of respondents by number of different regions frequented		Number of respondents by number of different regions frequented outside the Paris region	
	Number	%	Number	%
0	N/A	N/A	85	5.3
1	1232	76.1	1213	74.9
2	315	19.5	274	16.9
3	64	0.9	42	2.6
4	8	0.5	5	0.3
Total	1619	100.0	1619	100.0

Source: *Biographies et entourage* survey, INED, 2001

the places frequented is therefore to provide a completely different setting from that of the primary residence, be it on the coast, in the countryside or in the mountains. Almost 55 % of all respondents regularly leave the Paris region for family places in another region or country, in three quarters of cases to just one place (Table 9.10).

9.5 Conclusion

Data from the *Biographies et entourage* survey have enabled us to construct a geography of the family for Paris region residents aged 50–70. However, these inhabitants are by no means confined to the Paris region, as 85 % of them have links with other regions of France and other countries.

In this initial presentation of family territories based on *Biographies et entourage* data, we have examined respondents' reference spaces by making a distinction between places of origin, places defined in terms of the residences of living members of the respondent's descent group, and places actually frequented, including secondary residences. This set of places forms the family "map" of possibilities, which we have contrasted with the elective family territory identified by respondents as the places they regularly frequent, either because they live there intermittently or because they had a particular attachment to them at the time of the survey. Accordingly, by comparing this theoretical family map to the map of family places actually frequented by our respondents, we observe that over half of respondents have a real attachment to the places they visit where family members live or where they have bought or inherited a secondary residence. For two thirds of these respondents, this is the only family place they frequent. However, these percentages are an imperfect reflection of respondents' interactions with other locations in provincial France and abroad – be it to visit friends or to stay in hotels or on campsites, for example – as the present analysis concerns family ties only.

These results clearly show the importance of places in the way families function (weekly or monthly visits; help around the house; family get-togethers during the holidays; the role of the second home). Conversely, the way in which families configure their territories by clustering in one place or, alternatively, spreading themselves out in spatial terms – in other words, by making use of proximity and distance – is an indicator of the family ties that continue to exist in urban society, despite the individualization process that has marked recent decades.[17]

References

Attias-Donfut, C. (Ed.). (1995). *Les solidarités entre générations. Vieillesse, familles, état.* Paris: Nathan.

Bertillon, J. (1894). *Essai de statistique comparée du surpeuplement des habitations à Paris et dans les grandes capitales européennes.* Paris: Imprimerie Chaix.

Bonnin, P., & de Villanova, R. (Eds.). (1999). *D'une maison l'autre, parcours et mobilités résidentielles.* Paris: Créaphis.

Bonvalet, C. (1987). Les Parisiens dans leur maturité : origine, parcours, intégration. *Population, 42*(2), 225–247.

Bonvalet, C. (1991). La famille et le marché du logement. In M. Segalen (Ed.), *Jeux de familles.* Paris: Éditions du CNRS.

[17] Since the late 2000s, new research has been conducted on the family and space, notably with the data from the 2011 INSEE *Famille et logement* [Family and housing] survey which follows on from *Biographies et entourage*. It moves beyond the strict framework of the household to analyse the family and its territories, notably via the second home, be it a family home, a secondary residence or another regularly frequented place of residence. Imbert C., Déschamps G., Lelièvre E., Bonvalet C., 2014, "Living in two residences: mainly before and after working life", *Population & Societies* (INED) (507), http://www.ined.fr/en/resources_documentation/publications/pop_soc/bdd/publication/1666/

Bonvalet, C., & Lelièvre, E. (1995). Du concept de ménage à celui d'entourage : une redéfinition de l'espace familial. *Sociologie et société, XXVII*(2) pp.177–190.
Bonvalet, C., & Maison, D. (2007). The family circle: Spatial proximity and personal affinity. In C. Bonvalet, A. Gotman, & Y. Grafmeyer (Eds.), *Family, kinship and place in France* (pp. 27–68). London: Southern Universities Press.
Bonvalet, C., Gotman, A., & Grafmeyer, Y. (Eds.). (2007). *Family, kinship and place in France*. London: Southern Universities Press.
Chevalier, L. (1950). *La formation de la population parisienne au xixe XIX siècle*. Paris: INED.
Chevalier, J. (1974). Espace de vie ou espace vécu ? L'ambiguïté et les fondements du concept d'espace vécu. *L'espace géographique,* 1 pp.68–84.
Courgeau, D. (1975). "Le concept de migration" dans *Migrations, état civil, recensements administratifs,* actes du IVe colloque de démographie africaine (pp. 27–32). Ouagadougou, 20–24 janvier 1975, Institut national de la statistique et de la démographie.
Courgeau D, 1980. *Analyse quantitative des migrations humaines*. Masson, Paris.
Di Méo, G. (1990–1991). De l'espace subjectif à l'espace objectif : l'itinéraire du labyrinthe. *Espace Géographique,* 4.
Dubost, F. (1998). De la maison de campagne à la résidence secondaire. In F. Dubost (Ed.), *L'autre maison. La résidence secondaire, refuge des générations,* Autrement, 178.
Dureau, F. (2002). Les systèmes résidentiels : concepts et applications. In J.-P. Lévy & F. Dureau (Eds.), *L'accès à la ville : les mobilités spatiales en questions*. Paris: L'Harmattan.
Frémont, A., Chevalier, J., Hein, R., & Renard, J. (1984). *Géographie sociale*. Paris: Masson.
Gokalp, C. (1978). Le réseau familial. *Population, 33*(6), 1077–1094.
Gotman, A. (2007). Géographies, migrations and générations. In C. Bonvalet, A. Gotman, & Y. Grafmeyer (Eds.), *Family, kinship and place in France* (pp. 69–133). London: Southern Universities Press.
Gotman, A., et al. (2007). Variations saisonnières de la vie familiale : enquête sur les secondes résidences. In P. Bonnin & R. de Villanova (Eds.), *D'une maison l'autre, parcours et mobilités résidentielles* (pp. 177–212). Paris: Créaphis.
Imbert, C., Deschamps, G., Lelièvre, E., & Bonvalet, C. (2014). Living in two residences: Mainly before and after working life. *Population & Societies,* INED, 507. http://www.ined.fr/en/resources_documentation/publications/pop_soc/bdd/publication/1666/
Laslett, P. (1972). *Household and family in past times*. Cambridge: Cambridge University Press.
Lebras, H., & Goré, C. (1985). *Géographie physique et sociale de la famille dans la France actuelle,* CNRS Éditions, ATP Famille.
Lelièvre, E., & Imbert, C. (2002). L'entourage des Franciliens de 50 à 70 ans s'étend au-delà des limites de la région. In *L'atlas des Franciliens,* IAURIF/INSEE.
Lelièvre, E., Bonvalet, C., & Bry, X. (1998). "Event history analysis of groups. The findings of an on-going research project" New methodological approaches in the social sciences. *Population, An English Selection, 10*(1), 11–37.
Minodier, C., & Rieg, C. (2004). Le patrimoine immobilier des retraités. *Insee première*, 984.
Ortalda, L. (2001). *Le système d'entraide au sein de la parenté : entre logiques sociales et pratiques familiales*. PhD thesis, université Paris-X Nanterre.
Pinson, D. (1988). *Du logement pour tous aux maisons en tous genres*. Paris: PUCA, coll. Recherches.
Pourcher, G. (1964). *Le peuplement de Paris : origine régionale, composition sociale, attitudes et motivations*. Paris: INED, coll. Travaux et documents,43.
Remy, J. (1995). Multiplicité des lieux et sociabilité englobante. *Cahiers de sociologie de la famille,* 1.
Rosental, P.-A. (1993). *Espace et identités en France au XIXe siècle,* thesis defended at EHESS.
Roussel, L., & Bourguignon, O. (1976). *La famille après le mariage des enfants. Étude entre les générations*. Paris: INED, coll. Travaux et documents, 78.
Willmott, P. (1987). *Kinship and urban communities past and present*. Victorian Studies Centre, University of Leicester.

Chapter 10
The Contribution of a Longitudinal Approach to Family Solidarity Surveys: Reflections on the Temporality of Exchanges

Marianne Kempeneers, Éva Lelièvre, and Catherine Bonvalet

Since the 1980s, the topic of intergenerational family solidarity has been the focus of unprecedented interest among researchers, in the public arena and among family support services. In Europe in particular, this topic has become a real social issue, as attested by the numerous studies centred on the bonds that unite generations and the dynamics of family solidarity through time. The notion of *time* is thus central to this field of research and inevitably involves demographics. This is why we propose here to identify the major methodological challenges raised by the concept of "family solidarity" in twenty-first century demography. To do so, we will start by enumerating the various longitudinal perspectives observed in family solidarity surveys; we will then identify the context of temporal solidarity defined by each approach and we will offer methodological avenues that seem to hold promise for the future.

10.1 Overview of Family Solidarities: State of the Art in Research

As far back as the 1960s and 1970s, anthropologists and sociologists who studied the relational and support networks of their contemporaries stressed the importance of the bonds and exchanges among kin or extended families in an industrial society. It is not by chance that the first important writings on the topic appeared in Western Europe, where population ageing is more acute than in North America (Young and

This article first appeared in the journal *Canadian Studies in Population*, 34(1), pp. 69–83.

M. Kempeneers
Département de sociologie, Université de Montréal (UdM), Quebec, Canada

É. Lelièvre (✉) • C. Bonvalet (✉)
Institut national d'études démographiques (INED), Paris, France
e-mail: eva@ined.fr; bonvalet@ined.fr

C. Bonvalet, É. Lelièvre (eds.), *Family Beyond Household and Kin*,
INED Population Studies 6, DOI 10.1007/978-3-319-24684-0_10

Willmott 1957; Allan 1978; Pitrou 1978; Roussel and Bourguignon 1976). In the United States and in Canada, a few researchers approached the question very early on (Litwak 1965; Adams 1968), but most studies date from the early 1990s (Fortin 1987; Wellman 1999; Bengtson and Roberts 1991; Dandurand and Ouellette 1992; Godbout and Charbonneau 1996). In Europe, several important surveys confirmed the existence of bonds that unite generations (Bonvalet et al. 2007; Attias-Donfut et al. 1995; Attias-Donfut 2000) even if the relationships maintained by adult children with their parents are very diverse, and sometimes even ambivalent or conflictual (Finch and Mason 1993). Moreover, researchers in many countries have been working in collaboration to compare the dynamics of solidarity in these countries in order to better harmonize social welfare policies across the European continent (Bonvalet and Ogg 2007). Five major findings have emerged from these studies:

(a) *Family solidarity is maintained over time* despite the ever-growing shift toward nuclear families and individualization in our society. Only the modalities vary: contact modalities (frequency and circumstances) and the exchange of goods and services (lending of money, babysitting, provision of accommodation, home care and support, emotional support and care for sick, old or disabled persons). These contact and exchange modalities vary according to residential and affective proximity. They also vary by gender (women are more active), generation (the "pivotal" or "sandwich" generation is more heavily solicited), and social status (in low-income households, familial support may be preferred over public services due to economic constraints).
(b) *This solidarity is increasingly expressed on a vertical axis*, which means that more contacts and exchanges are observed between generations (parents/children/grandchildren) than between collateral relatives (brothers/sisters).
(c) *The family tie is highly specific*, creating a situation whereby the services exchanged among kin noticeably differ from the forms of support provided by public services, especially in terms of availability, diversity, permanence and cost (Pitrou 1987; Dechaux 1996). Furthermore, it has been observed that this bond leads to a kind of flexible reciprocity, often deferred in time and functioning as a sort of "insurance scheme" over the long-term but quite vague and with no guarantees (Coenen-Huther et al. 1994; Godbout and Charbonneau 1996; Déchaux 1996). Gift and counter-gift relationships bind individuals to one another, as opposed to mercantile relationships where the exchange ends as soon as one party repays its debt. "Within families, debts are not repaid once and for all, but maintained over years". These kinds of specific reciprocity in familial environments imply that family members must each be simultaneously considered in their role of both donor (or "caregiver") and of donee (or "receiver").
(d) *Norms of obligation are created and adjusted over time.* If we consider a gift as an exchange that serves a relationship, the relationship itself then becomes an arena for creating a sense of obligation, in the sense of "being obligated to". Relationships are thus built in a context of norms based on mutual expectations. Some think that obligation primarily arises in relationships that are established over time, the product of the interactions more than the result of external and imposed norms. For others, this normative system built up within familial and

intergenerational relationships over the life course is reinforced by historically and socially constructed norms. This said, the independence norms are also very widespread, and familial support operates more as a "safety net" than as a systematic resource.

(e) *Family solidarity is more intensely mobilized during critical events in the life course:* events such as births, conjugal breakdown, unemployment, illness, loss of independence in old age are all likely to mobilize support from the family circle.

The concept of "family solidarity" that emerges from these findings brings in a notion of *time*, as well as a concept of *exchange* (of goods and/or services), both of which are associated with the awareness of a shared sense of belonging that creates *bonds of reciprocity* and *norms of obligation*. Three distinct temporal aspects should be considered: *historical time*, which applies to the maintenance of solidarity over time despite structural change in both families and society; *generational* time implied by the primacy of "vertical" exchanges (intergenerational); and finally, *biographical time*, which refers to the calendar of individual and family trajectories, to the critical stages that require the mobilization of family solidarity and to the alternating caregiver and receiver roles played by family members. It is the interaction of these three temporal aspects that constantly creates and recreates the social landscapes where family solidarity is played out, in ways which vary according to the configuration of family models and to the alternatives offered by work environments or neighbourhoods and by the public authorities at different times in history.

10.2 Available Methods for Observing Temporalities

The following empirical observation methods can be used to collect temporal data:

(a) *Cross-sectional observation*: a situation is observed in its most complex modalities at a specific moment or at key moment(s). Cross-sectional observation offers insights into *historical evolution* by comparing observations collected at different times and, to a certain point, into *intergenerational temporality* when the interactive roles of several generations are described.

(b) *Longitudinal observation*: this may be conducted individually or by cohort, retrospectively or prospectively.

- Life event history data is often collected from subjects in a retrospective manner (like the life stories recorded in qualitative studies). In the field of family solidarity surveys, combining data on different aspects of the life course, this type of observation is most often qualified as biographical. It offers insights into the evolution of solidarity over the course of *biographical* time.
- In the case of panel follow-ups, prospective longitudinal observation is rarely individual. It provides a good method for studying *historical evolution* by comparing observations made during successive periods on the same sample. As the sample ages, the *generational support cycle* can be observed, with individuals moving from the role of the child to that of the parent, etc....

10.3 Why Time Must Be Brought into the Question

What are the preferred observation modes in the different family solidarity surveys?

10.3.1 Cross-Sectional Observation and the Different Time Patterns of Support

The first studies of family solidarity were primarily cross-sectional, the aim being to establish the scope of the family network and the permanence of kinship relationships (Roussel and Bourguignon 1976; Gokalp 1978), and to identify actual exchange practices (Pitrou 1978).

About 10 years later, another cross-sectional survey – the *Proches et parents* (Close friends and relatives) survey conducted by INED (Bonvalet et al. 2007) – marked an important step in the emergence of the question of time and of the changing patterns of support and needs. This survey had a triple objective: to describe kinship, to understand the network of the local family circle and to analyse the support system. Three kinds of support were identified: daily support at the time of the survey, exceptional support during difficult times in the past and finally, recurring support during the course of adult life (housing or employment). Three temporalities are thus explored in the *Proches et parents* survey.

10.3.2 Capturing Complex Temporalities by a Complementary Qualitative Approach

To complement the *Proches et parents* survey, about 100 semi-structured interviews were conducted on family and residential trajectories. The topic of support is included but is not central to the questions and was analysed in a PhD thesis whose conclusions shed light on the need to see support as a process: "Detailed data analysis has enabled us to make an in-depth study of support that emphasizes the broad scope of solidarity established between individuals and their local family circle. We observe that in contemporary families, it is rare to find someone who has neither given nor received support. Support is the norm of kin relationships. However, this investment is not unilateral, since in practically all families it is based on mutual exchange: each individual both gives and receives. Furthermore, the acts of support are not isolated events or actions: they are part of a process that unfolds over the life course" (Ortalda 2001).

These qualitative interviews demonstrated how the longitudinal approach can contribute to the analysis of these support networks and confirmed that the support network evolves over the life course. In early life, individuals receive from their parents. In the next stage, support is exchanged primarily between members of the same generation, and later on, support is essentially directed at one's children while support to friends, brothers or sisters is reduced. In fact, siblings are clearly more often in competition with the respondent's children than with his/her friends.

10.3.3 A Fuzzy Temporality

Though respondents readily describe the support they have either received or given, in the *Proches et parents* survey, they do not explicitly mention the temporality of the exchanges. But this vagueness is central: by not specifying the time when support was given or provided, these men and women thus ensure that the resources of their networks remain accessible to them at any time. They deliberately place themselves in a state of "ambiguity", support being a potential relationship that unfolds over time. The analysis of the interviews confirms that acts of support, far from being perceived as specific moments in one's life, are accumulated and reactivated along the life course. The existence of support then becomes the product of a bond established over time, and addressing varied needs.

10.3.4 Cross-Sectional Exploration of the Intergenerational Component

Another way of capturing the longitudinal dimension of support is to survey three generations at the same time, such as in the CNAV *Trois générations* (Three generations) Survey (Attias-Donfut 1995) which focuses on the dimension of filiation and genealogy rather than on that of the conjugal or residential family unit. It takes into account the importance of the generational lineage, accentuated by the increased mean length of life, and the advent of the multigenerational family. This survey is unique in this field of research, not only because it samples three adult generations of the same family by asking identical, symmetrical or complementary questions to each interviewed member, but also because of the generational structure, anchored in the pivotal generation, whose key role was thus highlighted for the first time.

10.3.5 Setting Up Large Panels: Prospective Longitudinal Analysis of Behaviours in a Sample of Households

Yet another way to capture the temporal dimension of support without asking retrospective questions or interviewing different generations of the same families is to create a panel comprising several modules; some of which are carried forward from year to year while others vary from 1 year to the next. This solution has been chosen by the United States since 1992 with the *Health and Retirement Study (HRS*) which concerns only the elderly, by northern Europe countries such as Norway, Belgium, Netherlands and England (with *ELSA*). However, in some instances, questions relating to support networks sometimes involved only one module on any given year, such as in Luxembourg. In Norway, the first wave started in 2002 (the first results have just been issued). The panel that gives some hindsight is that of Belgium, which took place over 10 years from 1992 to 2002.

With regard to panels, international surveys are in the process of replacing national surveys. One such example is the GGS *Generations and Gender Survey*, the first wave of which took place in 2004/2005, with a second one planned for 2007. The SHARE *Survey of Health Ageing and Retirement in Europe* is another.

10.4 Combining Relevant Temporalities: The Biographical Approach

Two recent surveys have broached the topic of family solidarity from an innovative angle: *Biographies et entourage* [Life event histories and entourage] by INED (2000) and *Biographies et solidarités familiales au Québec* [Life event histories and family solidarity in Quebec] by the University of Montréal (2004). Both have the following in common:

- They captured the historical importance of lineage combined with changes in the contact circle, beyond the individual life course.
- They examined change in terms of the changing position of individuals over generations, another way to explore the intergenerational component beyond the various time patterns of support.
- And finally, they integrated both qualitative and quantitative approaches.

10.4.1 The Biographies et entourage *Survey*

Though the *Biographies et entourage* survey was not specifically designed to address the question of family solidarity, the principles of data collection that were used captured many aspects of intergenerational solidarity.

The *Biographies et entourage* survey charts the familial, residential and occupational history of 2,830 Ile-de-France inhabitants aged between 50 and 70, and their entourage. The notion of entourage in this survey includes not only the family members going back four generations, (blood relatives and relatives by marriage) but also all the people with whom the individual has resided as well as other people, related or not, who have played a key role in the respondents' lives. The concept of entourage thus extends beyond the strictly intergenerational and familial dimension of the above-mentioned surveys (Lelièvre and Vivier 2001).

Once this framework of individual interactions had been defined, the objective of the *Biographies et entourage* survey was to follow changes in the respondents' entourage over their life courses by reconstituting its composition, its geographic distribution and the level of co-residence between its members. It was thus possible to reconstruct the composition of the network in terms of generations, territorial boundaries and its evolution over time; the great majority of people interviewed having each been a child, a grandchild, a parent and then a grandparent in turn.

Though the *Biographies et entourage* survey did not collect data on the various kinds of support exchanged among the entourage during the respondents' life course, indicators can nevertheless be established on the basis of frequency of contacts, geographical distance and affective closeness. It was thus possible to analyse the local or semi-co-resident function of the parent-child relationships (Bonvalet and Lelièvre 2005a), family territories (Bonvalet and Lelièvre 2005b) and the cross-solidarity between respondents aged 50 and 60 and their children and surviving parents (Bonvalet and Lelièvre 2005c).

Finally, the *Biographies et entourage* survey offers a way of combining quantitative and qualitative approaches in a single data collection process. Efforts were thus particularly focused on devising a questionnaire that encourages a conversation more similar to an open interview than the usual question-and-answer routine of quantitative surveys, but that still calibrates this dialogue in a closed questionnaire. Listening to the respondents' interviews provided confirmation of this narrative tone. This represents an intermediate method between a purely objectifying approach aiming to chart life courses independently of the meaning given to them by respondents and, at the other extreme, the approaches that focus on individuals' own interpretation of their lives (Coninck and Godard 1989). Though we often, wrongly, associate objective data with quantitative data collection and subjective data with qualitative data collection, Daniel Bertaux (1997) reminds us of the declarative character of the answers in both cases and points out their limitations, a fact confirmed by the results presented here.

10.4.2 The Biographies et solidarités familiales au Québec *Survey*

The *Biographies et solidarités familiales au Québec* survey, closely based on the principles of the *Biographies et entourage* survey, goes one step further, comparing, over time and three generations, a similar life period with multiple opportunities for family solidarity (birth and early childhood). Large quantities of data were collected on the kinds of support and exchanges identified during that period. Though less systematically, other critical moments were also investigated from the perspective of family solidarity opportunities, such as the loss of independence of ageing parents, periods of occupational uncertainty and other periods identified by the respondents as "difficult moments" in their lives (Kempeneers and Vanbremeersch 2002; Kempeneers et al. 2005a, b, 2006).

The objective of this survey, conducted in the Island of Montréal in the summer of 2004, was to analyse the changes in family solidarity in Quebec over three generations, in relation to the transformations in the family, in employment and in public policies. Thanks to the pioneering data collection methodology borrowed from the *Biographies et entourage* survey (multidimensional event history questionnaire), *Biographies et solidarités familiales au Québec* reconstructs the familial, occupational and residential life courses of 500 individuals born in Quebec between 1934 and 1954, along with those of their parents and their children. Three temporal dimensions are mobilized here: biographical, intergenerational and historical.

The approach chosen in the *Biographies et solidarités familiales au Québec* survey makes it possible to:

(a) Reconstruct the most important bonds woven over the respondent's life course
(b) Distinguish between family bonds and "close" bonds (friends, neighbours) and hence examine the specificity of the family bond in relation to support
(c) Position the entire process along the historical timeline of changes in the family, employment and public support policies.

10.5 Twenty-First Century Challenges for Demographers in the Field of Family Solidarity

This overview of the various ways of collecting temporal data on exchanges among family members pinpoints three major challenges for the demographers of tomorrow: (a) to promote experimental research in the field of quantitative data collection; (b) to develop collaboration with researchers who favour qualitative methods; (c) to pursue avenues for multi-disciplinary dialogue.

Quantitative data collection is a very particular field of experimentation. In some way and paradoxically, demographers are the victims of the costs incurred by quantitative data collection methods because they are the privileged analysers of public statistics (which are not experimental) yet at the same time, due to financial constraints, they are rarely the designers of quantitative data collection methods. Note, however, that this is not the case in countries with inadequate public statistics (developing countries), which would indicate that research conducted in the South is worthy of special attention. Moreover, demographers are often associated with public data collection, but the constraints are such and the framework so rigid that research on quantitative data collection tools must be conducted elsewhere. Nevertheless, it is thanks to this partnership that the science of public statistics evolves.

It is also necessary to develop a more active collaboration with researchers who favour qualitative methods, not only by undertaking qualitative follow-up after quantitative surveys (and not everybody does so) but by also integrating qualitative approaches in the entire development process of the quantitative method and in the questionnaires themselves (Lelièvre and Vivier 2001).

And finally, it is of primordial importance to pursue avenues for pluridisciplinary dialogue on the theme of family solidarity, since it is thanks to long years of research conducted in anthropology, history and sociology that our understanding of the dynamics of intergenerational exchanges has been enhanced. The demographic approach to these phenomena is, after all, relatively recent and, faithful to the legacy of anthropology, it has always assumed a dual quantitative/qualitative identity. These disciplinary affinities must be cultivated at all costs in the future.

References

Adams, B. N. (1968). *Kinship in an urban setting*. Chicago: Markham.

Allan, G. (1978). *Sociology of friendship and kinship*. London: Allen and Unwin.

Attias-Donfut, C. (Ed.). (1995). *Les solidarités entre générations. Vieillesse, famille, États*. Paris: Nathan.

Attias-Donfut, C. (2000). Rapports de générations. Transferts intrafamiliaux et dynamique macro-sociale. *Revue française de sociologie, 41*(4), 643–684.

Bengtson, V. L., & Roberts, R. E. L. (1991). Intergenerational solidarity in aging families: An example of formal theory construction. *Journal of Marriage and the Family, 53*(4), 856–870.

Bertaux, D. (1997). *Les récits de vie. Perspectives ethnosociologiques* (Collection Sociologie 128). Paris: Nathan.

Bonvalet, C., & Lelièvre, É. (2005a). *Le fonctionnement local des relations parents enfants*. Paper presented at the 25th conference of the International Union for the Scientific Study of Population, Tours, France.

Bonvalet, C., & Lelièvre, É. (2005b). Les lieux de la famille. *Espaces et sociétés*, La famille dans tous ses espaces, 1–2/2005, pp. 99–122.

Bonvalet, C., & Lelièvre, É. (2005c, June). Relations familiales des personnes âgées. *Retraite et société*, Les nouvelles données démographiques, 45, pp. 44–69.

Bonvalet, C., & Ogg, J. (2007). *Measuring family support in Europe*. London: Southern Universities Press.

Bonvalet, C., Gotman, A., & Grafmeyer, Y. (Eds.). (2007). *Family, kinship and place in France*. London: Southern Universities Press.

Coenen-Huther, J., Kellerhals, J., & Von Malik, A. (1994). *Les réseaux de solidarité dans la famille*. Lausanne: Éditions Réalités sociales.

Dandurand, R. B., & Ouellette, F.-R. (1992). Travail des mères, garde des enfants et soutien de l'entourage dans trois quartiers montréalais. In R. B. Dandurand & F. Descarries (Eds.), *Mères et travailleuses. De l'exception à la règle* (pp. 129–162). Québec: IQRSC.

De Coninck, F., & Godard, F. (1989). L'approche biographique à l'épreuve de l'interprétation. Les formes temporelles de la causalité. *Revue française de sociologie, 31*, 23–53.

Déchaux, J.-H. (1996). Les services dans la parenté: fonctions, régulation, effets. In J.-C. Kaufmann (Ed.), *Faire ou faire-faire? Familles et services* (pp. 39–54). Rennes: Presses Universitaires de Rennes.

ELSA (English Longitudinal Study on Ageing). http://www.ifs.org.uk/elsa/

Finch, J., & Mason, J. (1993). *Negotiating family responsibility*. London/New York: Tavistock/Routledge.

Fortin, A. (1987). *Histoires de familles et de réseaux*. Montréal: St-Martin.

Godbout, J., & Charbonneau, J. (1996). *La circulation du don dans la parenté. Une roue qui tourne*. Montréal: INRS- urbanisation.

Gokalp, C. (1978). *Le réseau familial*. Paris: INED, Population, 6.

HRS (Health and Retirement Study). http://hrsonline.isr.umich.edu/
Kempeneers, M., & Vanbremeersch, M. (2002). *L'Enquête-Pilote "Biographies et entourage" au Québec*. Rapport d'activités présenté au Ministère de la famille et de l'enfance au Québec.
Kempeneers, M., Vanbremeersch, M., & Van Pevenage, I. (2005a, May). *Pour une approche biographique des solidarités familiales au Québec*. Paper presented at the ACFAS conference, Chicoutimi.
Kempeneers, M., Vanbremeersch, M., & Van Pevenage, I. (2005b, May). *Les solidarités à travers les générations: qui est présent au moment de la naissance des enfants?* Paper presented at the conference of CSSS Nord de l'Île et St Laurent "La famille et les relations intergénérationnelles", Montréal.
Kempeneers, M., Vanbremeersch, M., & Van Pevenage, I. (2006, May). *Lieux de vie et entourage familial au Québec*. Paper presented at the ACFAS conference. Montreal: Univ. McGill.
Lelièvre, É., & Vivier, G. (2001). Évaluation d'une collecte à la croisée du quantitatif et du qualitatif, l'enquête 'Biographies et entourage'. *Population, 56*(6), 1043–1074.
Litwak, E. (1965). Extended kin relations in an industrial democratic society. In A. Shanas & G. F. Streib (Eds.), *Social structure and the family: Generational relations*. Englewood Cliffs: Prentice Hall.
Ortalda, L. (2001). *Le système d'entraide au sein de la parenté: entre logiques sociales et pratiques familiales*. PhD thesis, Université Paris X, Nanterre.
Ouellette, F.-R., & Dandurand, R. B. (2000). L'anthropologie des parentés euro-américaines. *Anthropologie et Societes, 24*(3), 5–20.
Pitrou, A. (1978 and 1992). *Les solidarités familiales*. Toulouse: Privat.
Pitrou, A. (1987). Dépérissement des solidarités familiales? *L'année sociologique*, 3ème série, *37*, 207–224.
Roussel, L., & Bourguignon, O. (1976). *La famille après le mariage des enfants. Étude sur les relations entre générations*. Paris: INED/PUF, Travaux et Documents,°78.
SHARE (Survey of Health, Ageing and Retirement in Europe). http://www.share-project.org/index.php?page=Home&menue=1&sub=
Wellman, B. (1999). *Networks in the global village*. Boulder: Westview Press.
Young, M., & Willmott, P. (1957). *Family and kinship in east London*. London: Routledge and Kegan Paul.

MIX
Papier aus verantwortungsvollen Quellen
Paper from responsible sources
FSC® C105338

If you have any concerns about our products,
you can contact us on
ProductSafety@springernature.com

In case Publisher is established outside the EU,
the EU authorized representative is:
Springer Nature Customer Service Center GmbH
Europaplatz 3, 69115 Heidelberg, Germany

Printed by Libri Plureos GmbH
in Hamburg, Germany